DEFEAT CANCER NOW

A Nutritional Approach to Wellness
For Cancer and Other Diseases

Tamara St. John

Defeat Cancer Now: A Nutritional Approach to Wellness for Cancer and Other Diseases.

1st Edition: 2012

Revision: 2018

2nd Edition: 2025

Published by Lake Front Publishing LLC

ISBN 13: 979-8-9924673-0-7

Table of Contents

Dedication

I would like to thank God for healing me and helping me to finish this book, which will glorify him and help millions of people. I believe that God will put this book in the hands of millions of people, so they can heal naturally using God's Pharmacy.

This book is dedicated to the many people who have battled cancer and won and also to those who unfortunately lost their battle. I would also like to thank my parents for helping me during my times of poverty, so I could afford food to help me stay healthy and alive. I will never forget those wonderful people that I have met along the way who unfortunately lost their battle with cancer; they touched my life dearly and will forever live in my heart.

"I can do all things through Christ who strengthens me."
Philippians 4:13 NKJV

Required Disclaimer

I am not a medical doctor and any information given within these pages is strictly for informational purposes only. I do not give medical advice but merely supply information for people to increase their knowledge base and conduct further research for themselves. Please consult with your physician before undertaking any alternative treatment as it could affect the profits of the pharmaceutical companies, physicians, hospitals, and insurance companies and then they would be highly upset if you weren't contributing to their billions of dollars in annual profits and keeping them driving their Mercedes and living in their mansions.

It is known that any undertaking or experimentation of alternative medicine is to be done of your own recourse, and I am not liable for damages. This book is merely an account of my own experimentation and how I healed myself of cancer; with God's amazing grace, using only alternative methods. By writing this account, I am utilizing my freedom of speech, freedom of press, and freedom of religion as protected by my first amendment rights in the United States Constitution.

All of the treatments I utilized are guaranteed under my freedom of religion; as I follow the bible for God's law on how to eat, which in turn reversed my cancer using God's pharmacy. "Worship the Lord your God and His blessing will be on your food and water. I will take away sickness from among you". Exodus 23:25.

Neither the treatments in this book, the statements made, nor the verses in the Bible have been evaluated by the FDA. It is imperative that if you fear that you have cancer that you consult with a qualified physician. This book will lay the foundation for which you can achieve Optimum Health through God's Pharmacy. God Bless.

Prologue

As I am climbing to the top of Mt. Baldy, in Southern California, in 70-80 mph winds and a 40-degree wind chill in the late spring, I am reminded of my cancer battle. As I struggle to make it up the mountain without being blown over the side, I wonder which was tougher, the cancer or this mountain? Of course, having and healing cancer has thrown me for a loop, and it was much more of a struggle to survive for a longer period of time than just the 3 hours it took to climb the tallest mountain in Los Angeles County at 10,064 feet. Yet still, climbing mountains feels a lot like cancer to me as it is always a struggle to reach the top or the path of wellness, but it is so worthwhile once you get there.

Life certainly isn't easy and has thrown me more than my fair share of blows along the way but what I have learned from this experience is to let go of the arrogance, embrace humility, have a helping spirit, trust in God, and always strive to reach the top of any obstacle.

I am not a doctor by any means, but I am just one of many who have conducted thorough research about natural healing and alternative cancer therapies. In the last few years, I have studied chemistry, biology, human physiology, epidemiology, biochemistry, and nutrition, all in an effort to educate myself about the properties of cancer cells and how to reverse cancer using only nutrition.

During the process of experimenting on myself I have written this true account of the ups, downs, and progress that I have encountered. Through God's divine guidance and my own experimentation, I found my true calling and have been healed of cancer. Yet I know that keeping cancer at bay and staying healthy will always be an ongoing process for the remainder of my life.

This book is an in-depth look into the world of alternative cancer therapy and natural treatments and is not meant to diagnose, give medical advice, or treat anyone. However, in writing this truthful account of my life and in my quest to heal my own health issues, I have managed to become a better person and ended up stepping into the destiny for which I have been so eagerly praying and searching.

I had planned for a much different life than this, don't we all. Life never seems to go according to our plans, but Gods plan for our lives always wins out. Unfortunately, I had to battle cancer in order to find my purpose in life. Now, if it were up to me, I would never have been sick to step into my reason for being. However, life just isn't fair and the sooner you realize that the better off you will be. Get past the "Why Me" and just accept what is and do something to fix it. I do enjoy helping and motivating people, and I hope that through my own experimentation and reversing cancer naturally, that I can inspire at least one person out there to have hope, keep fighting for their life, and to faithfully trust in the Lord for complete healing.

God has brought this disease into my life as a blessing, so I can share with you what I had learned, and hopefully save someone else in the process. It has also taught me to be humble, to be able to endure pain and discomfort, and to grow and live for your dreams while you still have the chance.

All and all, it is up to God as to when it is time for our demise and apparently God still has a plan for me to help others and I pray that I fulfill his plan for my life. In the process, I stepped into my destiny of helping others through telling my own story and hopefully giving other people hope into their own wellness plan. You can achieve Optimum Health through God's Pharmacy. Good Health and Blessings to all of you.

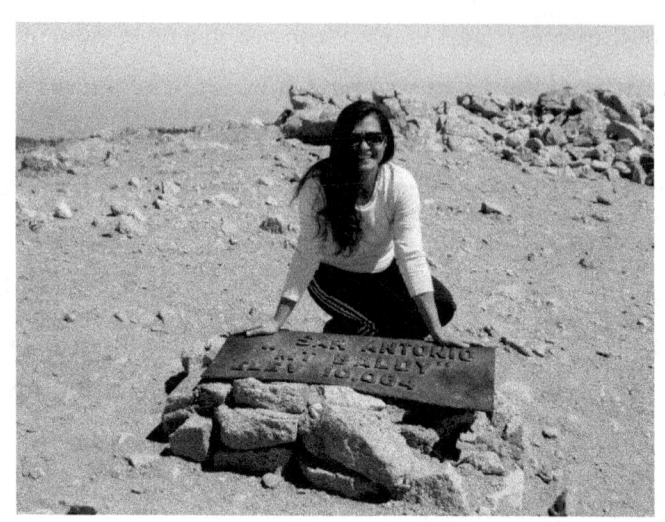

Me on Top of Mt. Baldy, CA. (Elevation: 10,064)

Chapter 1

My Cancer Story

When I started this book in June of 2009, I was indifferent to whether I would still be living by my 40th birthday in September. Oh, don't get me wrong; I wanted to live and was interested to see how my life would turn out. But I am not sure what is in the cards for me in the near future. Is anyone really?? Nobody really knows what the future holds, and every day is a gift and should be treated as such. As the saying goes; Life happens when you are busy making other plans. I am about to share with you how I came to diagnose myself with various types of cancer, how I treated them with various alternative methods, the affirmation of cancer, the test results, and the highs and lows that I had encountered through my personal experimentation in healing cancer naturally.

A little about me; my name is Tamara St. John. I am not a doctor, but someone who is highly educated and knows how to research an issue and solve problems effectively. I enjoy hiking, ice skating, traveling, zoos, museums, and generally anything new and exciting. I currently have a master's degree in business administration with a dual concentration in Accounting and Finance. I am also an Adjunct Professor at a college in Southern California, where I teach accounting and financial management. I grew up in Southern California and had ventured on many different career paths while I was completing my education. I have always been looking for the perfect career that I would enjoy doing, where it wouldn't feel like work, and where I could help others. I never could have imagined that this was where I would end up or that having cancer would be the catalyst that propelled me into my destiny.

In the beginning stages of cancer, I had the symptoms but didn't recognize them until much later. Sometime in 2008, I noticed that I was always tired and didn't know why. I don't just mean the tiredness that you feel when it is time for bed; I am talking about being completely dragging and needing to sleep about 12 hours a day. I just didn't have the stamina and energy that normal people my age had. If I went out to do something for a few hours, I would have to come home and nap for three hours just to feel better. I had felt completely drained and lethargic after only a couple of hours of activity, and I would feel this way throughout the day.

I had also noticed that my hair had begun to thin out drastically. I used to have very thick, long hair that hung down to my butt and then it started to thin out and I would lose a lot of hair in the shower daily. At the time, I had just attributed the hair loss to hormonal changes from aging and just shrugged it off.

I had also felt a few lumps under my chin that were hard and cyst like. I remember joking with a colleague at work that I probably had throat cancer and would die because I had no insurance. Due to the fact that I was only a part-time employee with no medical insurance and no money, I never went to the doctor to get any of the symptoms checked. I knew then that something was wrong, but I ignored the beginning warning signs.

In hindsight, I realize that all of these factors were the beginning warning signs that something was seriously wrong within my body. It wasn't until a year later that the other major symptoms of cancer began to appear and that is when I really began to worry.

A year after noticing the slight health issues, I was becoming more lethargic and exhausted. I still needed to nap every day, but now it was a four-hour nap between work, school, and homework. I also felt as if I was in a cloud or "brain fog" where I would have a hard time concentrating and always felt tired, even though I was sleeping twelve hours per day.

By April of 2009, I found a small lump in my left breast, and it was painful to touch. Knowing full well that my mother had breast cancer before the age of 40, I was a bit alarmed. But, since I did not have health insurance and not enough money to pay for any treatment, I decided to just pray about it. Of course, at this time, I was also a month away from completing my master's in business administration degree. So, I had to put my health on the backburner and concentrate on finishing my degree first. So, I just kept an eye on the small lump, kept ice skating, and kept to my gluten free diet.

At the beginning of May in 2009, I noticed several moles around my collarbone that had changed shape, changed color from brown to black, and started to crack and bleed. I had begun an all-natural topical treatment for skin cancer at that point, not knowing for sure that it was skin cancer, but knowing that those were the signs of skin cancer.

A few days later, I was terminated from my job, after three years, where the manager said that; "it just wasn't working out". As I was being fired, I smiled at the manager and said Thank you. I knew it would all be ok because I would be graduating in a couple of weeks and I already had two Universities interested in obtaining me as a part time professor.

A week after my termination, the lymph nodes underneath both of my underarms had swelled to abnormal levels. I had approximately five swollen lymph nodes underneath each armpit. Most of the swollen lymph nodes were the size of a kidney bean, but one lymph node was swollen much larger than the others and was the size of a couple of large grapes put together and was visible. The swollen lymph nodes were extremely painful, and I felt a throbbing, painful discomfort throughout the day and while trying to sleep. The deep, throbbing pain spread across my entire chest area, starting from underneath one armpit and going across my entire breast area, and finishing in the opposite armpit.

At this point, I also had quite a few lumps or cysts that had formed on my throat and one of them was large and visible. I had felt the lumps in my throat a year before, but they were smaller, and I had chosen to ignore them at the time. These lumps or cysts were hard and formed directly under my chin going all the way down my throat. This was also accompanied by a severe sore throat, making it hard to swallow, that had lasted on and off for over a year. I attributed this to twenty-two years of smoking and was thinking that it could be some type of throat cancer forming but wasn't sure. Whatever it was, I knew that the lumps didn't belong there and that the various symptoms that I was experiencing were not normal.

I still had to try to put all of these health issues to the back of my mind and stay focused on my pending final exams and graduation. Most people might have completely freaked out at this point, but I somehow maintained composure, although I honestly don't know how I did it. God was definitely with me then and now.

On the day of my last final exam, I had a telephone interview with the Employment Development Department (EDD); where they informed me that my former employer was fighting against paying me unemployment benefits. My former employer had lied to the EDD and said that I had abused students and went against company policy. Of course, I was dumbfounded since the manager had only said that "I wasn't working out". So, now I am thinking that I am going to be in for a lengthy lawsuit because I will be suing for defamation of character.

Due to my former employer lying about me, I had to complete a telephone interview with the EDD to determine my eligibility for unemployment benefits. The telephone interview was scheduled and had transpired about two hours before my last final exam to complete my degree. I got off the phone with the EDD and began to cry and hyperventilate, my heart was pounding through my chest, or possibly I was just having a major anxiety attack. I could not understand why all of these problems were coming against me all at once. I had to drive to school, crying all the way, hysterical. I still had to manage to pull myself together to pass my final and get my degree. It wasn't easy!!

So, I had managed to graduate with my M.B.A. and had great hopes for my future. I know that when God closes one door that he opens a window, and I know that when life comes at you the hardest is when you are closest to stepping into your destiny. I therefore knew that because of everything that has happened thus far, my life's path would somehow be great!!

Since I had managed to graduate, I was now able to focus upon my health and attempt to find a way to heal the various cancer symptoms that I was experiencing. After finding all of the lumps on my throat, lump on my left breast, swollen lymph nodes underneath both armpits, constant throbbing pain, brain fog, and misshapen moles on my body, I was very fearful and figured that I was going to die.

I was afraid because I didn't have any significant amount of money, no health insurance, and I was as brainwashed as the rest of the population into believing that cancer is a death sentence unless you utilize the traditional western medicine approach of surgery, chemotherapy, and radiation. It is frightening when you discover that you have a deadly disease and feel that you have nowhere or nobody to turn to for help or comfort. It was a very lonely, desolate time and God was my only savior in my time of need, so I turned to him.

At the point of finding the cancer and realizing what it was, I felt as if I would die. I figured that if I was going to die anyways, that it would be on my terms. After all, I believe that the Lord is in control of everything. I believe that God has a big book in heaven, and he already knows how and when each of us is going to die. Knowing that God already has my end date written in his big book, I figured that it didn't matter whether I was in a hospital or at home.

If I were going to die of cancer, it wouldn't include chemotherapy, mutilating surgery, radiation, needles, hospital visits, or doctors. I figured that if God had meant for me to die of cancer, then it wouldn't matter where I received treatment, and I chose to die at home. Conversely, if God wanted me to live, then he could save me no matter which treatment I had chosen.

I will never forget the day in June of 2009, when I had sat in front of the computer, crying out to God, and asked for God to lead me to whichever alternative treatments would heal me of the cancer within my body. I was immediately led to two different alternative methods for cancer, one of which I began immediately. I started The Budwig Protocol immediately because it was the most cost effective and easiest method to put into practice. Within a couple of weeks, I added in a few other protocols to my cancer arsenal to make up the "Defeat Cancer Now" plan. These were apricot kernels, juicing, detoxification, enzyme therapy, sunlight, and exercise.

After beginning all of the various alternative treatments, I began to experience extreme nausea, profuse sweating, hot & cold spells, dizziness, vomiting, and diarrhea. The reason that I experienced this healing crisis was due to doing all of the alternative treatments within an hour of one another. This "healing crisis" happened for a few days in a row until I figured out that I needed to spread out all of my alternative treatments throughout the day, instead of doing them all within an hour. I realized that I was detoxing from cancer too quickly and all of these signs were indicative of an overabundance of toxins attributed to cancer leaving the body.

Within a few months of beginning all of the alternative protocols for cancer, I had experienced a rash around my neck in the form of a ring. The rash was very itchy and uncomfortable all day long. I had begun to research the rash by interviewing others, who had experienced the same type of rash, and I had found that the rash I had was indicative of a cancer rash; known as, the Epidermal Growth Factor Receptor (EGFR), which is prevalent in advanced cases of HER1 type cancers. The EGFR rash was a good sign that cancer was detoxifying from my body. I had spoken to other cancer survivors, who also had experienced the EGFR rash, and they had verified that the rash would not subside until all of the cancer was out of my body. It took over 7 months, from October of 2009 to April of 2010, for the rash to finally dissipate.

It took almost a full year to successfully reverse the cancer, and I began to feel better by April of 2010. This is where I began to relax and quit most of my alternative cancer treatments and reverted back to bad eating habits, going back on the birth control pill, and drinking heavily. HUGE Mistake. I reverted back to my old ways and the cancer came back by November of 2010, which eventually landed me on my death bed by December of 2010.

When the cancer came back, it was in the form of lumps on my throat again, so I went back to utilizing The Budwig protocol to heal my cancer a second time. At this point, I slept up to 20 hours a day and was in constant brain fog. At the time, I didn't realize I was making a fatal error, which landed me close to death by the end of December of 2010. It is only with divine intervention that I am still alive to write this account.

It was a couple of days after Christmas, in 2010, and I had felt my body dying as I was lying on my couch. I was crying and had prayed to God that I was too tired to detox my body from cancer any longer and I was giving up, I basically told God that; "if he wanted me to live, he would have to detox the cancer from my body himself, because I was done." I then got up from the couch and went to bed. The next morning when I awoke, I had to run to the bathroom four times with extreme diarrhea. By the third time in the bathroom, I had felt the brain fog lift from me like a shade being pulled up on a window. I had realized that I was miraculously healed by God, enough to regain some of my energy, and by the beginning of January of 2011; I had enough energy to begin a detoxification regimen to rid myself of cancer once again.

Unfortunately, my body had too many toxins from terminal cancer, and I was detoxing my body too fast, which released many of the toxins back into my body, causing other health issues that needed to be healed. Throughout 2011 and 2012, I had been working on detoxifying my body of all of the accumulated toxins, from terminal cancer, that have caused such issues as extreme intestinal permeability, severe allergies with histamine reactions, boils, low thyroid, insulin resistance, high cortisol, depression, irritable bowel syndrome, ulcerative colitis, liver toxicity, and extreme weight gain.

By March of 2012, I was interested to see where I stood with cancer, even though I am still facing health issues in other areas. At that point, I had taken the Navarro urine test to determine how much cancer I have in my body and the test came back positive for cancer, most likely showing remnants of the breast cancer, I had previously. Although the cancer was still present in March, it was not life threatening at that point and was only a small amount in comparison to the amount of cancer I had previously.

Now, I did not take the Navarro urine test for my benefit because I could already feel that I still had trace amounts of cancer due to the "brain fog" I felt, which is different than that of someone experiencing brain fog from chronic fatigue syndrome, depression, or Epstein Barr. Those of you who have had advanced cancer know what I am referring to. I did the Navarro urine test to quiet the "haters" who kept sending me hate mail because I didn't have an "official" diagnosis from a medical doctor trained by the pharmaceutical companies. I will explain in a later chapter the scientific validity and significance of the Navarro urine test to detect cancer.

Now I am sure many of you are wondering how I knew it was cancer without an "official" diagnosis from a traditional, western medicine type doctor? Well, in the beginning stages, and symptoms I experienced in 2008, I didn't know it was cancer, but I had an idea. It wasn't until the cancer advanced to a point where it was abundantly obvious. Not to mention that when I began my alternative treatments for cancer, I was experiencing extreme detoxification symptoms and the Epidermal Growth Factor Receptor (EGFR) rash, indicative of HER1 type cancers. If someone doesn't have cancer in their body, there will not be an EGFR rash OR the extreme detoxification symptoms that I had experienced.

Now, it is highly possible that the cancer began somewhere else in my body, other than in my left breast. Most HER1 type cancers that include the EGFR are found in non-small cell lung cancer cases, but they can also be found in some advanced breast cancer cases as well. Since the lump on my left breast was visible and it had spread to my lymph nodes, I concluded it was indeed breast cancer.

Since I had other lumps, in other areas of my body, it is possible that cancer started there and moved to the breast tissue, I will never know. It is also possible that cancer could have started in my lungs, since I was a smoker of 22 years, and spread to the breast. Again, I will never know. In a way, I am glad I didn't have a traditional diagnosis because I am guessing that the cancer was far more advanced than I realized. Also, traditionally trained medical doctors are notorious for instilling fear in a patient, so they can begin surgery, chemotherapy, and radiation immediately.

I compare the diagnosis to a cold; everyone knows when they are coming down with a cold. You usually experience sneezing, a runny nose, and an overall feeling of ill will. The majority of people don't need to run to the doctor to get diagnosed with a cold to know it exists because all of the symptoms are obviously present. It is the same premise when the symptoms of cancer become overwhelming; there is no denying its existence.

In an ideal world, I would have gone to a doctor in 2008, when the lesser symptoms began, and found out when the cancer was only a stage 1 or 2, before it spread to the lymph nodes. However, in that case, I would have been as scared as anyone and been brainwashed into having my body parts removed. So, I believe it was a blessing that I didn't have health insurance or any money because it kept me from being pulled into the western medicine mantra of surgery, chemotherapy, and radiation. Instead, it forced me to think outside of the box and trust in the Lord that he would lead me to the correct alternative therapies to heal me.

As of this writing, I am still detoxifying my body to get all of my organs and hormones back to normal working order and get rid of the systemic candida that had caused the cancer in the first place. I will be discussing systemic candida as the cause of cancer in another chapter.

By November of 2012, for the first time in over three and a half years, the brain fog had finally lifted, and the lethargic feeling is gone. Although I am still healing intestinal permeability and other health issues, I can feel that cancer is no longer an issue in my body. Those of you who have had advanced cancer know the feeling that I am speaking about, but it is like coming out of a cloudy fog and being able to see clearly once again.

This book will take you through my journey into the various stages of my cancer battle, which alternative methods I had used and am currently utilizing to heal cancer, the biochemistry of the cancer cell, the detoxification process and other alternatives for getting healthy in the process. I will also share with you the major mistakes I made in treating cancer, what I learned from those mistakes, and how my mistakes can benefit you.

In my quest to heal cancer and other health issues, I had become a better person and stepped into a career of helping others through my tragic circumstances. My hope for anyone reading this book is that you stay positive through your fight and turn your trust toward the Lord. I am hoping that this book will help at least one person to survive their fight with cancer and come out on top; to me that would be the ultimate reward.

Update; I am still alive in 2024, 15 years later, although it has been no cake walk, I can assure you. For those who have been following me for a while, you know my struggles after stage 4 cancer was advanced adrenal fatigue diagnosed by a doctor and cortisol testing. I had suffered with adrenal fatigue for years following cancer, then a respiratory condition of which I am still trying to heal, IBS, IBD, ulcerative colitis, leaky gut, multiple food intolerances and sensitivities, MTHFR, and the list went on and on and on. I visited over 30 doctors, many traditional and many who were chiropractors, naturopaths, acupuncturists, and massage therapists.

Nobody could tell me why I was still sick with so many different things and nobody was able to help me heal. Everything was stuck in my body, and it wasn't until around 2023 when I finally figured out that my body was stuck in fight or flight mode for the past twelve years. I finally managed to get my body out of fight or flight mode and then my body was able to begin detoxing again to heal. I will go into detail about my experience with fight, flight, and freeze mode and what I used to heal in an upcoming book I am working on.

Chapter 2

What Is Making You Sick?

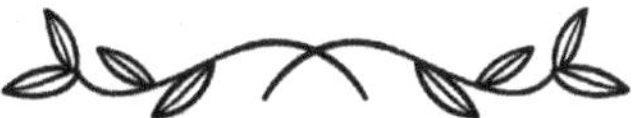

Ever since Richard Nixon declared the war on cancer in 1971, the cancer rates have skyrocketed to 1 in 3 women and 1 in 2 men, who will get cancer in their lifetime. Obviously, the current approved methods for treating cancer aren't working and America is the unhealthiest nation in the World. So, what has happened in the last 40 years and why are we getting sick?

The answer lies in many different avenues; chemicals, sunscreens, radiation, genetically modified organisms (GMOs) in the food supply, which is now being labeled as bioengineered ingredients, pesticides, antibiotics, drugs, alcohol, air quality, and chemicals in the water supply, just to name a few.

Everywhere you turn, you are bombarded with chemicals on a daily basis. Most of you probably clean your home with chemically laced products, which you inhale daily. You use toxic chemicals daily in your shampoo, conditioner, lotions, skin creams, makeup, cologne, perfume, candles, room spray, toilet cleansers, bathroom & kitchen cleansers, supplements, vitamins, hair dyes, hair products, and sunscreen.

All of these toxic chemicals, you inhale into your body or put them directly on your skin, which is your largest organ. Everything you put onto your skin soaks into your bloodstream, which can cause health problems in the future. Inhaling and putting toxic chemicals onto your skin daily may eventually lead to toxic overload, which can cause many health problems. Some of you may even have mold or yeast growing in your home and are breathing in those toxins as well.

Another toxic substance to be aware of is the pollution caused by chemicals dumped into our air and water. Pesticides and herbicides are sprayed onto the food supply, which permeates the soil and eventually runs into the water supply, poisoning plants, animals, wildlife, and sea life. It is known that these pesticides and herbicides are toxic to the body and contain cancer causing chemicals. How long do you think you can ingest these chemicals without getting sick yourself? The labels on all of these pesticides state that they are harmful if swallowed and to call poison control if ingested. If you won't go drink pesticides straight from the bottle that they come in, why would you ingest it on your food or in your water?

Chemicals, such as fluoride, have also been added to the water supply. Fluoride is a known carcinogen that can cause cancer. Chlorine is also added to the water supply, in order to kill bacteria, but ingesting chlorine can't possibly be good for the body either. According to the Environmental Protection Agency (EPA); "Exposure to excessive consumption of fluoride over a lifetime may lead to increased likelihood of bone fractures in adults and may result in effects on bone leading to pain and tenderness. Children aged 8 years and younger exposed to excessive amounts of fluoride have an increased chance of developing pits in the tooth enamel, along with a range of cosmetic effects to teeth." The EPA is admitting that excessive consumption of fluoride will lead to a variety of health problems. Of course, the EPA doesn't address all of the health problems associated with ingesting fluoride.

According to the EPA and reported by the Environmental Working Group; "there are over 316 known contaminants in our drinking water, with only 114 being regulated." Although, regulating the amount of chemicals that are safe for us to drink is ridiculous. No amount of toxic chemicals is safe for us to drink. But we aren't just drinking it, we are inhaling it in the shower, bathing in it where it soaks into our bloodstream, washing our clothes in it, and washing our food in it.

Now that you are up to speed on the chemicals found in everyday products, chemicals in the water, and chemicals in the air, let's take a look at what has happened to the food supply in the past twenty years and how our food is making us sick.

Genetically Modified Organisms (GMOs), the brainchild of Monsanto Corporation, are scientifically altered seeds to create a "bug resistant" superfood. Monsanto Corporation began tinkering with the food supply back in the mid-1990s; and since then, more people have had health issues with allergies, asthma, cancer, diabetes, inflammation, autism, celiac disease, rheumatoid arthritis, and a host of other health conditions.

I am not saying that GMOs cause any of these health conditions, but the rise of health problems, which directly correlate with the introduction of GMOs into the food supply, cannot be ignored. Could GMOs be the reason for the rise in health issues? I know, from personal experience, that there is a definite correlation between the foods you eat and the state of your health. It has also been proven, by many people who change their diet, that eliminating GMOs from their diet corrects many health conditions. In a future chapter, I have added a few testimonials from parents who have changed their families' diets; eliminating GMOs, and the positive effects they experienced.

Monsanto Corporation has been in the chemical business for many years, and they were the company directly responsible for creating DDT; a pesticide used from the 1940s through the 1970s, until it was banned in the United States by the EPA. Monsanto is also responsible for creating Roundup Ready pesticide for crops, which is highly toxic.

Monsanto is also responsible for Agent Orange, which is the chemical, known as Dioxin, which was sprayed on the residents and soldiers in Vietnam during the Vietnam War. I am sure that everyone has heard of the health problems of the Vietnam veterans and citizens who were in contact with Agent Orange (Dioxin) during the Vietnam War. If not, let me enlighten you; According to the Vets helping Vets website, "Symptoms of Agent Orange poisoning include cancer, birth defects, chloracne, severe personality disorders, liver dysfunction, gastrointestinal disorders, kidney problems, neurological damage, psychiatric problems, metabolic disorders, cardiovascular issues, vision problems, and loss of hearing." Many of the offspring of those residents were born without limbs or organs due to the toxic effects of Agent Orange.

Monsanto is also the company that is responsible for creating Recombinant Bovine Growth Hormone (Rbgh) and Recombinant Bovine Steroid (Rbst), which is a type of hormone and steroid that is injected into cattle and chickens, so they grow faster and are able to go to market quicker than the organic variety. Due to the amount of people getting sick, off of the hormones and steroids that transferred to the milk supply, Rbgh and Rbst were banned for use in the milk supply and now most milk product come from cows not treated with Rbgh or Rbst. Although Rbgh and Rbst are still used in animals and transfer to the non-organic beef and chicken you consume. All of these chemicals are known carcinogens and may cause cancer and other health issues.

Apparently, poisoning the air, water, and soil was not enough for this monstrous chemical giant. Since the advent of the many toxic chemicals created by Monsanto Corporation, they have entered into the food business by altering the genomes of the seeds of the plant, known as Genetically Modified Organisms (GMOs).

Here is an example of the way a genetically modified crop is altered to create a GMO. Let's take for example an ear of corn; the seed of the corn plant is spliced and mixed with fungicide, herbicide, pesticides, Agent Orange, bug parts, fungus, and mold and then put back together to grow a "super" corn that is supposedly able to withstand pests. Since the pesticide is injected directly into the plant itself, when a bug takes a bite of the food, their stomach explodes, and they die.

The problem is that the bugs have become immune to these GMO crops and the chemical companies now need to create "stronger" GMO crops by increasing the pesticides they use within the seed of the food plant, hence the reason for adding Agent Orange to the new breed of GMO corn. If all of these toxic ingredients implanted into our food can make the stomachs explode in insects, which feed off those plants, what do you think it is doing to you?

Since GMOs have been introduced in the 1990s, gastrointestinal disorders have skyrocketed, as well as a host of many other diseases. I am not directly blaming GMOs for the rise in gastrointestinal disorders or other diseases; however, I find the correlation of the introduction of GMOs and the rise of these disorders to be interesting enough to write about. I personally cannot eat any GMOs, Rbst, Rbgh, or any other food that has pesticides or chemicals because I have extreme allergic reactions to them. When you have gastrointestinal disorders, such as intestinal permeability, food allergies and intolerances will increase exponentially.

Due to the toxic overload from detoxing too fast from cancer, which created my intestinal permeability issues, when I have eaten any food with any GMOs, I will have a histamine reaction show up on my face within 10 minutes of eating any chemically laden food. The allergic reaction is so bad that it forms a giant cyst near my nose and swells to affect my eyesight and my mouth. Sometimes they come in the form of large boils.

Currently the list of GMOs includes Corn, sugar beets, cotton, zucchini, soy, Hawaiian papaya, alfalfa, and canola. GMO crops: such as corn and soy, are made into various derivative ingredients that are put into processed foods. A few of the GMO ingredients that you will find hidden in the ingredient list of your favorite processed foods are maltodextrin, soy lecithin, cottonseed oil, canola oil, whey, soy protein isolate, whey powders, high fructose corn syrup, corn syrup, corn sugar, aspartame, textured vegetable protein, soy sauce, tamari, NutraSweet, malt, soy milk, and many others.

Most recently, the term GMO is no longer utilized as much as it has been renamed "bioengineered ingredients." The term "bioengineered ingredients" is what you will see on many processed food items on the store shelves, but it is the same as GMOs, just re-labeled. If you are interested in finding out more about GMOs (aka; bioengineered) in the food supply and how to avoid them, I suggest visiting the Institute for Responsible Technology website for the most up-to-date information. You can find that information at www.responsibletechnology.org.

If you currently have health issues and are interested in healing yourself naturally, start with what you are putting in your mouth. Cut out all GMOs, processed foods, non-organic meats, sugars, sodas, and other chemically laced food products. Just by changing the way you eat and what you put into your body will make a huge difference in the way you feel and help to heal your body naturally.

Chapter 3

What is Cancer?

When people hear the word "Cancer", they generally think of death and sickness. Because I actually lived through cancer, and now know how it works, I choose to think of cancer as only nutrient deficiencies, parasitic and/or worm infestation, and fungal growth, all of which can be reversed through detoxification and the proper food choices. I first had to change my thinking that cancer was a death sentence and keep telling myself that cancer is only a nutrient deficiency like any other you might experience and take it from there. As I began to educate myself on nutrition, biology, physiology, biochemistry, and epidemiology, the more I learned about how a cancer cell works and the properties of cancer. I soon realized that cancer is indeed reversible, provided you detoxify your body properly and feed your body the proper nutrition.

After continuous research and experimentation on my own body, I have come to realize that cancer is only a symptom that your body is deficient in certain nutrients. The reason people get cancer is from an overabundance of toxins in the body, candida, parasites/worms, which all create an acidic condition. When the body is acidic, it can lead to nutrient deficiency because your body cannot absorb proper nutrients when it is bogged down with toxins.

In order to reverse cancer, you need to detoxify the body and introduce beneficial enzymes and nutrients that your body is lacking, and the cancerous symptoms will reverse on their own. What you are doing is removing the "root cause" of the cancer, so the body can heal itself. When you detoxify the body of all of the processed foods and toxins that have been ingested, you will be on the path to strengthening your immune system to be able to eliminate cancer and other diseases on their own. It sounds much simpler than it is, and it is not an easy process, but it can indeed be done.

Everyone develops cancer cells in some form or another at some point in their lives. However, some people have a pH (period of hydrogen) balanced body, where their immune system is working optimally, and can fight off cancer cells before they become dangerous and form into malignant tumors. Those people that have a highly acidic pH or have a highly acidic diet will most likely end up with cancerous tumors or other diseases. I know of people that can eat anything they want and still have a pH balance of 7 or better, unfortunately, I am not one of those people. If I were to eat anything that is acidic to the body, my body would become very acidic; I would become extremely lethargic, have no energy, and have to go to sleep for a few hours to a whole day until my body recovers.

After much research and experimentation, I have concluded that candida and parasites are at the heart of most, if not all, cancers and diseases. According to Dr. Tullio Simoncini, an oncologist, "there is only one cause of cancer: candida, which, according to the anatomical branch concerned causes different histological reactions. This is the reason why there are so many types of tumors."

Dr. Alan Cantwell states that "the cancer microbe exists in the blood and tissues of all human beings and animals. It is found in people who are healthy, as well as sick." According to Dr. Cantwell, "Cancer is pleomorphic, which means that it can appear in many different forms. These forms range in size from submicroscopic forms resembling viruses, up to the size of much larger forms resembling yeasts, fungi, and parasites."

Nobel laureate Dr. Johannes Fibiger of Denmark received his award for his discovery that a candida parasite is the cause of cancerous tumors. He had observed mice, in a sugar factory, which possessed cancerous tumors. Cockroaches in the same factory were feeding on the droppings of the cancerous rats; afterward they showed symptoms of the same candida parasitic infection. Dr. Fibiger then fed healthy rats the parasite infested cockroaches and the healthy rats harbored the same parasitic fungus cancerous tumors. I also find it interesting that mice which had cancerous tumors, were found in a sugar factory, since cancer and candida are both known to feed on sugar as its main fuel source.

Otto Warburg was born in 1883 Germany and grew up to be a doctor in Chemistry and Doctor of Medicine. Dr. Otto Warburg went on to be the director of the Kaiser Wilhelm Institute for Cell Physiology. Otto Warburg won the Nobel Peace Prize in 1931 for his discovery that cancer cells must have an anaerobic, meaning lack of oxygen, environment in order to thrive. When you have too many toxins, due to candida and parasitic infestation, blocking your cells from performing their duties, they become anaerobic. This basically translates into the fact that cancer cannot live in an oxygenated environment. Based upon Dr. Warburg's theory, it makes sense that if you open the cancer cell wall and oxygenate the cancer cell itself, the cancer will reverse itself.

Dr. Budwig speaks of a nutrient deficiency, namely, lack of omega 3's, to be a cause of cancer and other diseases. Obviously, if you have a fungal infection of candida albicans within the body, you will have problems absorbing the proper nutrients, which can lead to a nutrient deficiency of the cells. If you continue on the path of a nutrient deficiency for too long and the candida in the body continues to grow, cancerous tumors become a symptom of those deficiencies and fungus.

I believe that God had created our bodies to be self-healing if we feed ourselves the proper nutritious meals. However, with more and more people eating processed and fast foods, we have become a nation of increasing sickness and disease. Think about it this way, the United States is supposed to have the best hospitals and medicine in the world, but people are still becoming obese, sick, and dying in record numbers.

I believe that this downfall of health in the United States is directly related to the downfall of nutrition in individuals and the increase in reliance upon the healthcare system and pharmaceutical medication, as opposed to taking responsibility for your own health through healthier eating. This has become a processed world of fast food; where families no longer make the time to sit down at the table with one another and eat a homemade, nutritious meal, but instead opt to order a pizza, go through a fast-food drive-through, or microwave their meals. Making a nutritious meal is easy to make once you get the hang of it and usually takes no longer than 15 to 20 minutes to prepare an organic, wholesome meal for your family.

According to T. Colin Campbell, PhD and author of The China Study, "Our food choices have an incredible impact not only on our metabolism, but also on the initiation promotion, and even reversal of disease, on our energy, on our physical activity, on our emotional and mental well-being and on our world environment."

Another factor that may have contributed to the increase in disease and cancers may also be linked to Genetically Modified Organisms (GMOs) within the food supply. Almost all of the foods that you find on the traditional supermarket shelves contain genetically modified ingredients, hormones, steroids, preservatives, msg, additives, pesticides, chemicals, high fructose corn syrup, and many other harmful ingredients. All of these man-made ingredients are causing people to accumulate toxic waste that increase the likelihood of candida overgrowth and parasite infestation, both of which may lead to Cancer, Diabetes, Fibromyalgia, Heart Disease, Alzheimer's, Parkinson's, Multiple Sclerosis, Autism, ADHD, Rheumatoid Arthritis, High Blood Pressure, Obesity, Gout, and many other ailments. The majority of people will visit a doctor that prescribes them drugs, which will never heal the body, but which further harms the body and only masks the symptom.

Most people are conditioned to believe that cancer is a death sentence. However, cancer is just a way of your body telling you that your cells are lacking certain nutrients, oxygen deficient, and your body has an overabundance of toxic substances that need to be eliminated. In order to reverse the symptoms of cancer. In order to reverse cancer naturally, one needs to detoxify the root cause of cancer in the body, feed the cells proper nutrients and pump the cancer cells full of oxygen to reverse cancer and begin the healing process of transforming cancerous cells into healthy cells and ultimately a healthier body.

Chapter 4
Why You Haven't Heard of Alternative Methods

Alternative remedies have been in existence since biblical times, with the use of herbs, spices, and nutrition as a way to heal the body. Although back then, they weren't called "alternative" but just the everyday remedies that were known to work for every ailment. It is only within the last one hundred years that the medical monopoly really escalated into medical doctors being nothing more than over glorified, over paid drug dealers, pushing the latest pharmaceutical experiment on trusting, unsuspecting patients.

In the early 1900's, The American Medical Association didn't impose much of any regulation upon doctors or medical schools. Some doctors were even able to buy their degrees without having attended medical school. The majority of medical institutions were all teaching nutrition-based courses of healing, as part of the curriculum. So, what has changed and how did this medical monopoly come about? This is where the corruption of the medical establishment begins, with a few key corrupt individuals.

It all began with a man by the name of Abraham Flexner, who worked for The Carnegie Foundation in 1908. Mr. Flexner had devised a plan that the medical schools needed more oversight and control. Abraham decided that it would be a great idea to infiltrate the medical schools and make them all conform to one standard, refusing funding to those medical schools that didn't adhere to the new regulations in favor of a drug-based curriculum, as opposed to a nutritional based curriculum.

This is where all of the medical schools began teaching prescription drugs as a solution to mask the medical problem instead of healing it with nutrition. Even the medical books were completely re-written to eliminate any words of nutrition or its benefits to health. John D. Rockefeller and Andrew Carnegie provided financial backing to put The Flexner Report into action in 1910. Refusal of funding for medical schools immediately closed many institutions from 340 to 80 medical schools by 1940. It is easy to see how the entire medical establishment was strong armed into compliance by being threatened with closure.

According to T. Colin Campbell, "The problem with doctors starts with our education. The whole system is paid for by the drug industry, from education to research. The drug industry has bought the minds of the medical profession. It starts the day you enter medical school. All the way through medical school everything is supported by the drug industry."

In continuing with the suppression of healing cancer naturally; Dr. Otto Warburg, who was discussed in the last chapter, was ahead of his time and it amazes me that more people aren't aware of his work. Dr. Warburg's work is suppressed to keep people from knowing the truth. The same type of suppression had happened with other pioneers who knew how to heal cancer and disease naturally, such as Max Gerson, Dr. Johanna Budwig, Dr. William Kelley, Rene Caisse, and many others.

There are literally hundreds of alternative methods to heal cancer and other diseases naturally, but they are hidden from the public. When learning about these alternative methods, you will most likely find that western medicine and the pharmaceutical companies will laugh off alternative methods as quackery. It is clear that western medicine needs to try to discredit the alternative methods because they will lose billions of dollars in profit if people learn of their efficacy. There is just no money to be made from using God's Pharmacy, so the drug companies dismiss it as quackery.

Upon researching the various alternative methods to heal cancer, I had come across four protocols that I successfully combined to heal cancer naturally: Enzyme Therapy, The Budwig Protocol, Juicing Greens, and Laetrile Therapy. Along with these therapies, I also used exercise, sunlight, and detoxification as methods to help cancer heal quicker.

Now that you can see why alternative methods have been suppressed from the public, let's look at the treatment methods of western medicine. The problem with treating Cancer through the traditionally accepted methods of surgery, chemotherapy, and radiation is that they are rarely effective in the long term. Let's start with the faulty idea of surgical removal of a body part. If there is a tumor in the breast, removing the entire breast will not stop the cancer from spreading and may indeed cause it to metastasize to other areas of the body. Also, the reason that the tumor developed in the first place was only a symptom that something was wrong within the body. Western medicine treats the symptom by removing the tumor, as opposed to treating the original cause of the tumor. When you treat the original cause of the tumor, the tumor will retreat on its own. Your breasts did not cause your cancer, but your lifestyle, diet, or other factors caused cancer, which led to a tumor. The same goes for any other type of cancer. If you have brain cancer, do you remove the brain? NO. You shouldn't even need to remove the tumor from the brain, as any good alternative therapy will boost the immune system, which will reverse the tumor and cancer naturally.

The second part of the western medicine mantra for cancer treatment is chemotherapy and radiation. Chemotherapy and radiation are known carcinogens; meaning that they are toxic chemicals and toxic to the body, which is known to induce cancer. Chemotherapy and radiation eliminate the good cells in the immune system along with the cancer cells, so they leave no line of immune defense for the individual to fight off the cancer.

The goal of the western medical world is to eradicate cancer before the toxic treatment wipes out the immune system and kills the patient. However, we know that this isn't happening, as more and more people are dying from the treatments for cancer and not the cancer itself. I have seen it happen many times, where an immune suppressed patient goes into the hospital, only to be given toxic drugs that further suppress the immune system. What happens is that the patient will succumb to the illness because their immune system has been completely depleted. It absolutely makes no sense to give the body toxic chemicals, which cause cancer, to try to fight cancer. It makes much more sense to strengthen the immune system of the individual, so they can fight cancer on their own.

Statistics for cancer in allopathic medicine are faulty because the medical establishment only keeps track of patients for five years to determine whether or not the cancer treatment of chemotherapy and radiation was successful. This means that if the cancer returns after five years, as it usually does due to the toxic effects of chemotherapy and radiation, the medical establishment still considers their treatments to be a success. So, if you die one day after the five years of receiving the "approved" treatments for cancer, then the medical establishment chalks it up as a success. This is how the statistics are skewed in favor of the pharmaceutical companies and the toxic medicines they administer.

The actual success rate of chemotherapy and radiation, as a weapon against cancer, is much lower than ever reported. It is also known that research is rigged by drug companies. According to T. Colin Campbell, "Research and academic medicine merely carry out the pharmaceutical industry's bidding. This can happen because: the drug companies, and not researchers, may design the research, which allows the company to "rig" the study." It is clear to see how the pharmaceutical companies alter studies in favor of their toxic drugs.

Think about it, none of the medications you are currently taking have healed you of anything. Medications simply mask the symptoms but never get to the root cause of the problem. Alternative treatments, which are found in nature, will get to the root cause of the problem and can reverse most any condition. It just takes time and patience to figure out which plants, vegetables, seeds, nuts, spices or herbs are applicable for which condition or ailment.

Alternative methods for cancer aren't really the "alternative" because they are sourced from nature which have existed and been used since Biblical times. The chemical approaches of western medicine are actually the unnatural and often ineffective "alternatives". The problem is that the pharmaceutical companies cannot profit from treatments that are derived from nature. Since there is so little money to be made from nature's solutions, the drug companies harvest bountiful plants and biochemically alter them. Once patented, the drug is the property of the drug company for years before others can replicate their formula. As with any business, the fiduciary responsibility is to its owners and shareholders and exists to create profits.

It boils down to corporate greed, which found a way to profit from sick and desperate people. Presently, we are not given a choice of using nutritionally based methods that are much safer, to heal cancer. Instead, the pharmaceutical companies and the medical establishment label people as "quacks" if we choose to use God's Pharmacy over Man's Pharmacy. This is also the case if your child is diagnosed with cancer, you won't have the choice to treat your child with alternatives to heal as the medical establishment could report you as being a neglectful parent and report you to child protective services, which in turn could take your child away and force the "approved" cancer treatment on your child all without your permission. This proves that we are not living in a free country. We are not given the freedom of choice or the freedom of speech because we will be ostracized and sometimes prosecuted, if we use solutions outside those that are considered the "standard of care" by the medical establishment. What has happened in this country as far as the medical establishment and pharmaceutical companies are concerned is criminal, and a far cry from freedom.

Chapter 5
A Question of Genetics

I have heard many people exclaim that cancer is a genetic pre-disposition as is most other diseases. However, genetic predisposition to certain diseases can be altered using nutrition. For instance, there were people in my family who were alcoholics, and I had heard from when I was young that I must not ever drink, or I would be one too. Just putting that in the mind of a child or a child watching the alcoholic behavior of a parent or relative is an influence that the child would grow up and perpetuate because they know of no other upbringing. By detoxifying the body, cutting out all forms of sugar, and increasing magnesium, the craving for alcohol will go away. It is possible through proper nutrition and positive thinking that someone can alter their "so-called" genetic fate.

Let's look at Type 2 Diabetes. I have heard families exclaim that everyone in their family has diabetes; therefore, they will get it too. It is a self-fulfilling prophecy. Not to mention that everyone in a family with diabetes usually has very poor eating habits and they do not eat nutritious food. If a child grows up in an environment where the family is primarily living off of processed or fast food, the child will not have much of a chance to become healthy until they are old enough to make their own decisions regarding the type of food they want to eat. At that point, they have been conditioned since they were young to eat unhealthy foods and most adults continue the pattern of unhealthy eating, unaware that their poor choices are causing them to be sick.

The same was true for my family and it was told to me when I was young that my mother had breast cancer and therefore, I was at greater risk of getting it. Had I known then what I know now, I know that a genetic pre-disposition to disease does not always apply. You can have a genetic predisposition to having a naturally acidic or alkaline balanced body type, which can contribute to acquiring disease. However, this too can be rectified with a proper diet.

According to T. Colin Campbell, "…not all genes are fully expressed all the time. If they aren't activated, or expressed, they remain biochemically dormant. Dormant genes do not have any effect on our health." He goes on to state that diet and environment are what cause our genes to go into a dormant state. It has been proven that many cultures, which do not have high rates of cancer and disease, will succumb to cancer and disease if they migrate to another culture and adopt a western diet.

In a later chapter, I will go over the various types of foods that create acidity or alkalinity in one's body and how to eat properly. Proper nutrition is the basis for changing the pre-disposition of many diseases. If you change your eating habits and eat only foods that are high in alkalinity and balance your pH level, it is probable that you will never experience cancer, diabetes, or other diseases because your immune system and the oxygen level in your blood is killing disease before it is allowed to formulate in your body.

Therefore, the choices that we make as to the foods we eat and the foods we feed our families will directly impact whether we suffer with "so-called" genetic diseases or whether we remain healthy. T. Colin Campbell states, "…we can all optimize our chances of expressing the right genes by providing our bodies with the best possible environment-that is, the best possible nutrition." By starting your families on nutritious food choices, not laced with genetically modified organisms, hormones, steroids, antibiotics, preservatives, radiation from microwaves, and the like, you will be propagating a healthy behavior that can last for generations. Think of it, a healthy world where people no longer need doctors or medications for sickness because everyone is making healthy choices at the dinner table.

Chapter 6
Detoxification

The first step to healing cancer or any disease is to detoxify the body of the accumulated toxins, which is the root cause of the problem. A buildup of toxic sludge in the colon, gut, blood, and tissue will eventually lead to ill health and disease. Once you get to the root cause of the problem and remove the toxins within the body, the cancer can begin to heal itself.

Detoxification of the body will help to rid the body of the accumulated toxins that caused cancer or a specific ailment in the first place. In order for detoxification to be the most effective, it should be done in a certain order to make sure the channels of elimination are clear to release the toxins. During detoxification, you may feel sick, this is due to a Herxheimer reaction; also known as a healing crisis. You may feel as if you are coming down with the flu, but this will pass once the toxins are released from your body. During detoxification it is imperative to get plenty of rest and drink plenty of water to flush the toxins out of your system.

How do you know if you are toxic? If you suffer from any of the conditions and symptoms listed in the box, then you definitely need to detoxify your body. Granted, this is only a partial list as I may have missed some ailments that also need to be detoxified from the body. The proper order and various detoxification protocols will follow behind the toxicity list.

Symptoms of Toxicity

- Fatigue, Adrenal/Thyroid Failure
- Cold hands or feet
- Muscle Aches, Lupus, Joint Pain
- Chronic Fatigue Syndrome
- Neuropathy, Epstein-Barr Virus
- Overall Bad Feeling, Coughing
- Headaches, Migraines, Wheezing
- Poor Memory, Mental Fog, Depression
- Irritability/Anxiety, Mood Swings
- Insomnia, Hyperactivity, ADD/ ADHD
- Symptoms of Autism
- Vaginal Yeast, Vaginal/Rectal Itching
- Menstrual Problems, PMS Symptoms
- Endometriosis/Infertility
- Hormone Imbalance, No Sex Drive
- Cystitis/Urinary Tract Infections
- Prostate Irritation
- Indigestion, Protruding abdomen
- Eczema, Psoriasis, Athlete's Foot
- Cancer, Swollen Lymph Nodes
- Colds and Flu, High Blood Pressure
- Alzheimer's & Parkinson's
- Blood or Mucous in Stool
- Autoimmune diseases Sinus Infections, Post-Nasal Drip
- Ear Infections/Itching
- Respiratory Problems
- Asthma, Hay Fever, Allergies
- Heartburn/Acid Reflux
- Gas/Bloating, Diarrhea, Constipation
- Colitis, IBS, Crohn's Disease
- Leaky Gut Syndrome
- Ulcers, Intestinal Pain,
- Chemical Sensitivity, Dry Mouth
- Skin Rashes, Hives, Itching, Boils
- Rosacea, Dry Skin, Bad Breath
- Burning/Puffy Eyes, Dark circles
- Thrush (yeast in the mouth & throat)
- Fingernail/Toenail Fungus
- Over or Under Weight
- Low Blood Sugar (Hypoglycemia)
- Food Cravings (sugars & starches)
- Fibromyalgia, Rheumatoid Arthritis
- Over sweating, night sweats
- Diabetes, Acne, Cystic Acne
- Fluid retention
- Dark colored urine

Colon Cleanse

When beginning a colon cleanse, there are many different types to choose from. You can either use liquid Bentonite clay and Psyllium Husk taken daily and every evening or you may use a kit that is usually found in any vitamin or health food store. All of the colon cleanse kits will work differently because everyone's body chemistry is different, so it is difficult to say that one kit is better than another. The kits usually work when you take a combination of pills per day according to the instructions on the box.

I will sometimes opt for the detox kit, but I also utilize the liquid Bentonite Clay/Psyllium Husk method. With the Liquid Bentonite Clay, I take a couple of ounces of liquid Bentonite clay and follow it with an 8-ounce glass of room temperature water. The room temperature water helps to expand the liquid Bentonite clay in the system, which will soak up the toxins within the body. Liquid Bentonite clay is a negative ionic electrical charge, which attracts positively charged particles in the form of toxic poisons. Because the toxins in the body are positively charged and the bentonite is negatively charged, they are attracted to one another like a magnet. So, the bentonite clay will soak up the toxins and carry them out of your body through your stool.

I usually take a few ounces of the liquid bentonite clay with an 8-ounce glass of room temperature water and wait about an hour. I then take 2-4 capsules or 2 Tablespoons of psyllium husk with an 8-ounce glass of room temperature water. If you take the psyllium husk in powdered form, you must mix it into the water and drink it quickly, follow up with more water afterward. I will take this method at various times throughout the day and right before bedtime. Wait at least an hour before or after eating before taking this method or the vitamins and minerals from your food won't have time to assimilate.

The Bentonite clay will soak up the toxins in the body and the psyllium husk is a fiber that will bind and carry the toxins out of your body the next time you experience a bowel movement. Ideally, you should be experiencing 2-3 bowel movements per day, and you should not have to strain. If you are not experiencing 2-3 bowel movements per day, you are most likely constipated with toxic material in your colon and are in desperate need of a colon detox.

If you enlist the detox kit method of detoxification, follow the instructions on the box. If you enlist the liquid Bentonite clay/Psyllium husk method, then you want to continue it for about a week. This is where it is important to pay attention to your body and how you feel when you do this cleanse. The kit is usually safer for those who are new to detoxification.

While conducting the colon cleanse, you may notice black, tarry stool, mucoid plaque, mucoid rope, slimy mucous, parasites/and or worms coming out of your body. Don't be alarmed as this is a normal part of detoxifying the colon and the first step into bringing back good health. All of the sludge that has accumulated along your colon walls over the years will be eliminated and you will feel better once you are free from the toxic sludge that has taken up residence along your colon walls. After you have successfully completed the colon cleanse, it is time to move onto cleansing the body of a fungus known as Candida Albicans.

Candida Cleanse

Candida Albicans, often referred to as just "Candida," is a yeast like fungus that grows within the body and causes a host of health problems that manifests itself in various toxic symptoms. It is a common condition that approximately 85% of the population experiences, yet few know how to treat the underlying cause which is causing their symptoms.

Candida overgrowth can be caused from taking antibiotics, pharmaceutical drugs, birth control pills, sugary foods, starchy foods, foods containing gluten, processed foods, and stress. All of these will alter the balance of good to bad bacteria in the body, creating an overgrowth of Candida.

Many people suffer from conditions like eczema, psoriasis, cancer, acne, headaches, sinusitis, fibromyalgia, allergies, sugar cravings, alcohol cravings, inability to lose weight, yeast infections, bad breath, thrush, thyroid problems, hormonal imbalance, autoimmune disease, and many other conditions. If you experience any of these conditions listed above or any of the conditions listed in the "Symptoms of Toxicity" chart, it is highly likely that you have an overgrowth of Candida Albicans in your body.

In order to properly detoxify your body from candida and be on the road to good health, you must have completed the colon cleanse first to clear the channels of elimination. It is wise to change your eating habits to starve the candida of its fuel source while on the candida cleanse to achieve maximum efficiency. If you do not change your eating habits, you will continue to feed the candida and you will not be able to eradicate it from your body.

There are plenty of candida detox kits on the market that will help to eliminate candida. All of the detox kits will work differently depending upon the severity of the candida. Some people will have good luck with a candida kit if their candida isn't too severe of a problem. However, some people experience systemic candida, which is a more severe type of candida infection that is difficult to eradicate with just a candida kit, in which case you will need a more detailed detoxification regimen.

Various foods contain an anti-fungal compound which helps to get rid of candida naturally. The anti-fungal foods consist of garlic, leeks, onions, ginger, grapefruit seed extract, oregano, black walnut, and Pau D'arco. I personally like to use a clove of garlic, a hunk of ginger, 1 Tablespoon of Olive Oil, and 1 cup of Water all blended together and taken at night before bed. Another way to rid the body of candida is to make sure to include anti-fungal foods to your diet on a daily basis, use lots of garlic, onions, and oregano in your cooking.

It is also imperative to re-populate your body with good bacteria. When you have candida, the bad bacteria in your body outweigh the good bacteria, which is what is making you sick. Adding probiotics and prebiotics to your diet will also help to starve the candida from your body and balance the ratio of good bacteria to bad bacteria. Do not take the garlic/ginger mixture or a candida detox kit within 3 hours of probiotics or prebiotics to experience the best results. This is why I take the garlic/ginger mixture at night and then do the probiotics and prebiotics during the day and stop 3 hours before taking the garlic/ginger mixture.

Foods you cannot eat on a candida diet or while detoxing from cancer; no sugars, no starches, no processed foods, no high fructose corn syrup, no fruit, no dried fruit, no melons, no artificial sweeteners, no sodas, no fermented foods, no malted products, no alcoholic beverages, no yeasts, no breads, no cheeses, no vinegar containing foods or condiments, no gluten, no meat, and no antibiotics.

I have outlined a list of foods that you can eat while on a candida diet. It is good to stick to this list while you have Cancer as well, because fungus, such as, Candida Albicans, can also fuel cancer growth, as we discussed in an earlier chapter. So, by eating these foods, you can aid in eliminating candida and help to eradicate many health conditions.

Foods Allowed on the Candida Diet

CATEGORY	FOOD TO EAT	NOTES
VEGETABLES	Asparagus, Avocado Broccoli Brussel sprouts Cabbage, Cauliflower Celery, Cucumber Collard greens Eggplant, Garlic (raw) Kale, Leeks, Okra Onions, Peppers Radish Seaweed Spaghetti squash Spinach, Romaine Summer squash Swiss chard Tomatoes Turnip Zucchini	• Vegetables starve the Candida of sugar and mold that feed it. • Vegetables can absorb fungal poisons and carry them out of your body. • Avoid starchy vegetables such as carrots, sweet pota toes, potatoes, yams, corn, , and all squash except zucchini, beets, peas, parsnips and all beans except green beans. • Buy fresh vegetables and eat them raw, steam or grill them. Add a little garlic and onions for flavor as they are especially helpful with Candida. • If you steam the vegetables, drink the water that is left over, it contains most of the potassium and B vitamins that are

		cooked. • Eat at least 5-9 servings of vegetables everyday (a serving is ½ a cup). Thus, eat 2-5 cups a day. • Do not use any dressings on salads aside from fresh lemon juice and extra virgin olive oil.
LIVE YOGURT CULTURES	Plain yogurt Probiotics	• Live yogurt cultures (or probiotics) help your gut to repopulate itself with good bacteria. • The live bacteria in the yogurt will crowd out the Candida yeast and restore balance to your system. • Buy only plain yogurt that is Rbgh/Rbst free. Greek yogurt is a good choice, without any additives. • Yogurt from goat and sheep milk is even better, as they tend to contain fewer chemicals. • Good bacteria will also produce antifungal enzymes that can help you fight Candida.

PROTEINS	Beef Chicken Fish Eggs	• Proteins are almost completely free of sugars and mold, so they restrict the Candida. • Eat only fresh and organic meat. • Processed meat like lunch meat, bacon, smoked, vacuum packed, and spam, is loaded with dextrose, nitrates, sulphates and sugars and should never be eaten. • Eat only wild salmon, cod, sardines, and trout. No farmed or Atlantic salmon.
NUTS AND SEEDS	Almonds, Walnuts Cashews, Pecans Filberts, Brazil Pumpkin seeds Sunflower seeds	• Nuts & Seeds are a high protein food that starves Candida and restricts its growth. • Avoid peanuts and pistachios as they tend to have higher mold content and the peanut is not a nut, but a legume.

		• You can remove mold by soaking the nuts in water. Make sure the nuts and seeds are raw. • You can also buy pure nut butter, such as cashew and almond butter.
GLUTEN FREE GRAINS	Buckwheat Millet Amaranth Quinoa Wild and brown Rice	• Grains contain a high amount of fiber, excellent for keeping the colon clear. • Grains also act like a pipe cleaner in your intestine, grabbing nasty toxins, such as pollutants, chemicals, pesticides and heavy metals. • Make sure any grain is gluten free.

HERBS AND SPICES	Basil, Black Pepper Cayenne, Cilantro Cinnamon, Cloves Cumin, Curry, Dill Garlic, Ginger Nutmeg, Oregano Paprika, Rosemary Tarragon, Thyme Turmeric	• Contain antioxidants and anti-fungal properties • Increase circulation and reduce inflammation. • Improve digestion and alleviate constipation. • Most herbs and spices are beneficial in your fight against Candida. • They're great for livening up food if you're on a limited Candida diet.
OILS	Virgin Coconut Oil Olive Oil, Sesame Oil, Pumpkin seed oil Macadamia Oil, Almond Oil, Flax Oil, Safflower Sunflower, Coconut butter, Ghee, Organic butter.	• Use cold pressed oils and virgin oils. • Heating or boiling destroys many of the oil's nutrients. • Only Virgin Coconut Oil should be used for cooking because it retains its nutrients at high heats.

BEVERAGES	Water with lemon, Cinnamon Tea, Green Tea, Clove Tea, Ginger Tea, Chamomile Tea, Pau D'arco Tea, Peppermint Tea, Licorice Tea, Lemongrass Tea.	• All of these herbal teas have antifungal properties. • If you're missing your morning coffee, try Green Tea instead. • Adding lemon to the water helps to alkalize the body.

The candida cleanse can be performed at the same time as the parasite cleanse, which is discussed next.

Parasite Cleanse

Many people never realize that parasites can be living within their body and creating their health problems. Parasites consist of worms, roundworms, tapeworms, hookworms, and many other nasty invaders of the body which create many of the health problems you may be experiencing.

About 85% of people currently have parasites and/or worms living in their body and don't know it. You may have parasites if you live with animals, have eaten improperly cooked foods (i.e., sushi), have drank water from an unclean source, or have eaten any vegetables that weren't cleaned properly. If you suspect you may have parasites, you can do a parasite cleanse to rid your body of the nasty critters.

The parasite cleanse can and should be done in conjunction with the candida cleanse. You will need the following ingredients: Wormwood Capsules, Clove Capsules, and Black Walnut tincture. The wormwood and cloves will kill the eggs and larvae of the parasites, while the black walnut kills the live parasites.

The method of the parasite cleanse is to take 3 of the Wormwood capsules and 3 of the Clove capsules, 3 times a day for two weeks. That is a total of 9 clove capsules per day and 9 wormwood capsules per day. At the same time, take 20 drops of the Black Walnut tincture, mixed in water, 3 times a day for two weeks. That is a total of 60 drops of black walnut tincture per day. The black walnut tincture will also help to eradicate candida within the body as well as the parasites. You can opt to eat Black Walnuts in place of the Black Walnut tincture.

There are also parasite cleanse kits on the market which may be easier to do if you are new to detoxing. The parasite kits work the same as a colon cleanse kit or a candida cleanse kit, where you take pills or powders from a package specified by the directions on the box.

You can and should do parasite cleansing and the candida cleanse at the same time, or if you are really toxic, then do the candida cleanse first followed by the parasite cleanse. The reason for this is that you don't want to release too many toxins at once. All toxins pass through the liver, and you don't want your liver to become overloaded with toxins. So, if you feel like you need to do these cleanses separately, that will work just as well.

Parasites and worms are very tricky and often hide or become immune to certain ingredients. Therefore, it is good to take a short break between cleanses for about 5 days and then start up again. Vary the amounts of parasite cleanses, for instance, maybe do the black walnut, wormwood, clove mixture for 10 days and take a 5-day break, then switch to a parasite cleansing kit and complete it. Then take another short break and switch back to the black walnut, wormwood, clove method. Keep varying the Parasite cleanses so they don't become immune and die off.

Below is a picture of a two-and-a-half-foot dead ropeworm, being released through colon hydrotherapy. The second picture is of a rope worm that I had passed in 2016, after a negative parasite test. Traditional parasite tests that are through a lab will often only test for one or two types of parasites, so these comprehensive parasite tests are not very effective. You can still have parasites and worms even with a negative test, as in my case. I had to send the ropeworm I passed off to an independent lab to verify it was a ropeworm.

You could have these parasites and/or worms living inside of you right now and not even know it; therefore, it is so important to do a regular detox for parasites and worms.

After you have successfully completed the colon, candida, and parasite cleanses, you can move onto the kidney cleanse.

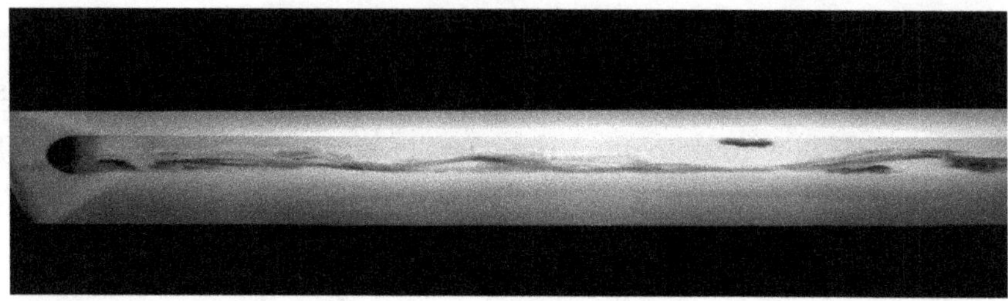

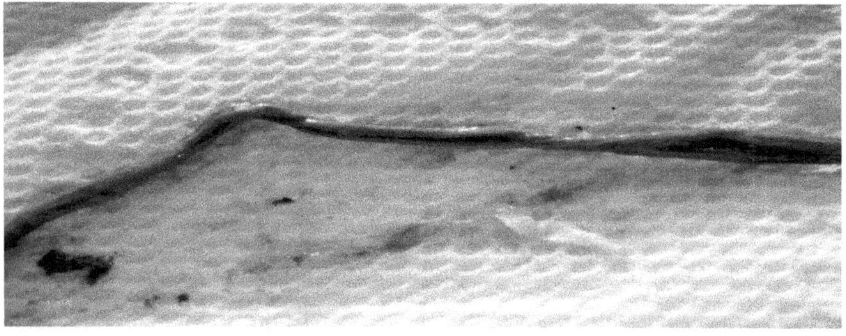

Kidney Cleanse

The kidney cleanse will help to rid the kidneys of kidney stones and will get the kidneys working efficiently. In order to cleanse the kidneys, you can brew tea made of parsley. Put 4 bunches of fresh parsley into a quart of water and bring to a boil. Let the mixture cool a bit and drink ½ cup of parsley tea daily for 3 weeks.

There are also teas on the market that are specifically designed for a kidney detox, which contain parsley and/or uva ursi and can also be used to aid in detoxifying the kidneys. You can also find kidney detox kits in a health food store.

Another way to cleanse the kidneys is to add parsley to your juicing regimen. You can also add dandelion greens which will also help to detoxify the kidneys as well. Below is a picture of kidney stones.

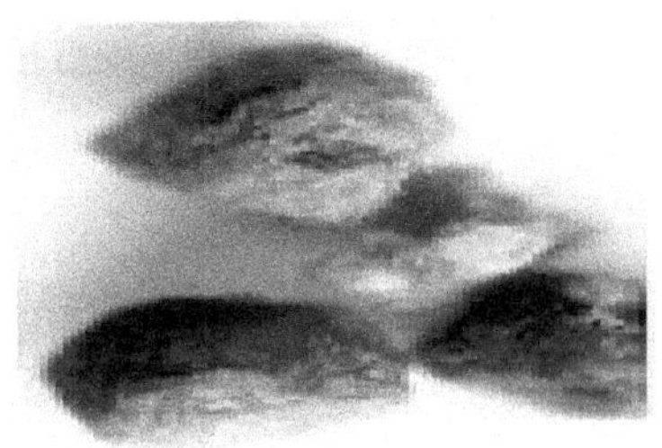

Liver Cleanse

Now that you have completed all of the other cleanses, you have cleared the channels of elimination to make way for the liver cleanse. The liver cleanse should be the last organ on your list of cleanses. Many people suffer from allergies, asthma, cystic acne, fibromyalgia, cancer and a host of other conditions. The reasons for these conditions are not only stemming from candida overgrowth but can also be related to an overabundance of gallstones which are clogging your liver. Even if you had your gallbladder removed, it is still possible to have gallstones clogging the liver. These stones that clog your liver will cause health problems and most all cancer patients have a clogged liver, so it is important to detoxify this organ.

You may also have gallstones clogging your liver if you have ever taken prescription medication, birth control pills, drank excessive amounts of alcohol, hepatitis, cirrhosis, taken illegal drugs, chemotherapy, radiation, or have or have had cancer. This cleanse is mostly from Dr. Hulda Clark, with a few additions to maximize the benefits, and works great but is exhausting. Make sure that you have nothing to do the evening and day after the liver cleanse, as you will be rather tired from performing this cleanse. It is very important that you do not jump to this cleanse, you MUST do the other cleanses in proper order, or the channels of elimination may not be clear to do this cleanse successfully.

Do not eat anything after 2pm the day you begin the liver cleanse. You will need Epsom Salt, Olive Oil, Organic Pink Grapefruit juice, Black Walnut tincture, Ornithine Capsules, and liquid Bentonite clay. At 2pm; mix together 3 cups of purified water and 4 Tablespoons of Epsom Salt in a large container. Put the mixture in the refrigerator to chill for the start of 6pm.

6:00 pm: Drink 3/4 cup of the Epsom Salt mixture.

8:00 pm: Drink 3/4 cup of the Epsom Salt mixture.

9:45pm: Mix 1/2 cup of Olive Oil with 1/2 cup of Organic Pink grapefruit juice and 20 drops of Black Walnut tincture into a glass jar with a lid. Take 8 Ornithine capsules with a glass of water. You can also take a melatonin to help you sleep if you don't think the Ornithine capsules will be enough. Visit the bathroom once more.

10:00 pm: Shake the mixture until watery and drink with a straw within 5 minutes, then immediately lay down on your right side with your right knee up to your chest. This will help the gallstones flow down the biliary duct. Sleep until 6 am.

6:00 am: Drink 3/4 cup of the Epsom Salt mixture. You may go back to bed.

8:00 am: Drink the last 3/4 cup of the Epsom Salt mixture.

10:00 am: You may now eat something but try to make it light.

When you visit the bathroom in the morning, you may see gallstones floating to the top of the toilet. The gallstones will vary in color and size depending upon your level of toxicity. The gallstones can be dark green, light green, or yellow in color. If you have passed any gallstones, you will need to repeat this liver cleanse once a month until all of the gallstones have been eliminated.

You didn't accumulate these gallstones overnight, so this process may take quite a few repeats to eliminate all of the gallstones clogging your liver. I had passed over 1,800 stones and it took almost 6 months of cleanses to do it. The Liver Cleanse will help you to eliminate allergies, asthma, have clearer skin, and other ailments for good.

A hint while doing this cleanse, when you start passing gallstones or right before, take a few ounces of Liquid Bentonite Clay with a large glass of lukewarm water. This will help to soak up any toxins that get re-released back into your body. When the gallstones start releasing from the liver, toxins can be re-released back into the body, and you want to avoid this so as not to cause further problems. This is a very important step and should not be skipped.

I had made a mistake while doing this cleanse, as I was repeating this liver cleanse every two weeks, instead of once a month, and not taking the Bentonite clay to absorb the toxins. What had happened is that I had re-released too many toxins back into my body and created other health problems, such as leaky gut syndrome, IBS, high cortisol, hormonal imbalance, low thyroid, and extreme weight gain. This is why it is important to only do this cleanse once a month and utilize the liquid Bentonite clay as a buffer to help in soaking up excess toxins.

In addition to adding the liquid Bentonite clay to this liver cleanse, it is a good idea to follow up with coffee enemas to flush out the additional gallstones, which didn't leave the body during the cleanse. I personally like to do three coffee enemas the day of the liver flush, after you have passed gallstones. And then follow up with two coffee enemas per day until you notice less gallstones floating in the toilet.

Another way to detoxify the liver is to take extra doses of milk thistle capsules, turmeric powder or capsules, Uva Ursi, beets, beet greens, and dandelion greens. You can add these to your daily juicing regimen or take them on their own. You can also find liver detox teas, liver tonics, and liver detoxification kits either online or at your local health food store. All will help to detoxify the liver in a more gradual manner.

Coffee Enema Liver Detox

The coffee enema will sound crazy to most people, as it did to me, until you learn about the history and benefits. I swore up and down that I would never do a coffee enema and then I broke down and did one and can't imagine a detoxification regimen without it, especially if you are trying to heal from cancer.

The benefits of coffee enemas were accidentally discovered in World War I, when a nurse in the hospital accidentally filled a soldier's enema bag with coffee instead of water. According to Dr. Lawrence Wilson, who quoted an article written by Gar Hildenbrand, in the Healing Newsletter in 1986, the story goes like this:

"The coffee enema may have been first used in modern Western nations as a pain reliever. As the story goes, during World War I nurses kept coffee pots on the stove all day long. The battle surgeons and others drank it to stay awake while working horrendously long hours. Enema bags hung around as some patients needed help moving their bowels. There was a severe shortage of pain medications. So, they were forced to save the pain drugs for surgical procedures with little or none for follow-up after surgery. When surgical patients woke up from operations without the benefit of further morphine injections they would scream in pain and agony from the surgery, and they would be constipated as well from the anesthesia drugs. For the constipation, a nurse was preparing an enema for constipation. Instead of fetching water for the enema, she accidentally dumped some cool coffee into the patient's enema bag, undid the release clamp, and into the patient it flowed." I'm not in so much pain," the poor soldier said. It was a coffee enema moment in history. Thus, began the use of coffee enemas to help control pain."

Since there was a shortage of pain medication in World War I, the hospital began using coffee enemas. Coffee enemas were even utilized for pain and written in the Merck manual, used by doctors, until the 1970's when the coffee enema and its benefits were taken out of the Merck manual. My theory is that doctors figured out that the coffee enema was detoxifying the liver and healing patients of cancer, pain, and other diseases to which their toxic drugs were no longer needed.

Dr. Max Gerson, who created the Gerson therapy for Cancer and other diseases, utilized coffee enemas to detoxify the liver and manage pain, for advanced cancer patients, along with fresh vegetable juices to heal the body naturally. The coffee enema works to release the bile from the liver, thus increasing glutathione and detoxifying the liver of harmful toxins. This liver detox is easy to do and is actually very relaxing once you get the hang of it.

You will need an enema bag; I bought mine at Wal-Mart for around $5.00. You must only use organic coffee because it contains no chemicals which are utilized during the processing of regular coffee. Organic coffee is very important because your colon will soak up whatever you put into it, and you do not want chemicals from regular coffee soaking into your body. Your goal is to get the toxins out, not put them back in.

To start the coffee enema, you will brew a pot of organic coffee with purified water (not tap water) and then let the coffee cool. I used to make the coffee at night before bed and then use it first thing in the morning after the coffee had cooled overnight. To do a coffee enema, fill the enema bag with the brewed room temperature, organic coffee and hang the filled bag a couple of feet above the bathroom floor. Lay a large towel down in the bathroom and get comfortable with something to read and a timer. Make sure to lie on your right-hand side, as this is the side where your liver is located. Use a little coconut oil or lubricant at the end of the insertion tip. Insert the tip and gently let a cup or two of coffee run into the colon. Stop the flow of coffee from the enema bag, if you feel too much pressure. Some people can hold more coffee and some less, this will take practice until you find what is comfortable for you.

It is a wise decision to do a quick enema first to get any fecal matter out of the colon first, which will make it easier to be able to hold the coffee enema for the full 15-20 minutes. Make sure to lie on your right-hand side because this is the side that your liver is on and will make it easier for the liver to release the toxins. The coffee enema should be held for at least 15-20 minutes, so the gallbladder will release toxins into the liver and the liver will then release its toxins by increasing bile flow. If you begin to cramp, you can take deep breaths, and the cramp will usually subside.

You can also massage the colon while performing the coffee enema. This will help to release any dried or old fecal matter that may be stuck within pockets in the colon. Don't feel bad if you can't hold it for the entire 20 minutes the first few times, this takes practice. Through experimentation, I have noticed that I can hold more coffee when I have done a quick enema first or when I haven't ingested enough water throughout the day and am dehydrated. Because your colon soaks up what you put into it, if you are dehydrated, it will soak up the water from the coffee. This is why it is imperative to use only filtered or bottled water when brewing organic coffee.

The more you perform this cleanse, the easier it will become. In time, you will be able to feel and hear the noise of the gallbladder releasing into the liver, which sounds like a gurgle or burping noise. The coffee enema can be done a few times a day but make sure that you are drinking vegetable broths or fresh vegetable juices after the enemas to replace any minerals lost. You can also eat a banana to replace the issue of depleted potassium levels.

As you can see, there are quite a number of various liver cleanses. Start slowly with the liver cleanses as if you do a liver cleanse too fast it will release too many toxins back into the system which will cause other issues to deal with after you get rid of cancer. Try the different types of liver cleanses to see which one works best for you.

Glutathione & The Liver

I have already discussed a bit about glutathione and the liver in regard to the benefits of coffee enemas, but what exactly is glutathione and how does it detoxify your liver?

Glutathione is the master detoxifier of the liver and gallbladder. You cannot get glutathione from a pill or a patch, but your body has to produce it from the foods you eat. Although there are many companies out there that will try to sell you a glutathione pill or a patch, they are a waste of money, in my opinion. I discussed in the previous section the benefits of the coffee enema and how it increases glutathione production to the liver, which aids to detoxify the liver.

Another great way to increase glutathione production within your body is through turmeric, milk thistle, whey protein powder, and dandelion. You can also increase glutathione production through an amino acid known as L-glutamine, which also helps to heal intestinal permeability (aka; leaky gut syndrome). The various foods that help to increase glutathione production within the body are avocado, whey protein, eggs, l-glutamine, turmeric, milk thistle, and dandelion.

I usually take turmeric by the teaspoon, mixed into a glass of lukewarm water and drunk down quickly. I found I save a lot of money by buying my turmeric in bulk from an Indian grocery store, as opposed to buying turmeric supplements. Through my experimentation, I noticed that by ingesting turmeric; to increase glutathione production, it helps to break up gallstones naturally, aids in repairing intestinal permeability, heals boils & cystic acne, and heals irritable bowel syndrome quickly.

Juice Fasting

Another method of detoxifying the body is through a juice fast, where you give your digestive system a rest and subside on nothing more than freshly prepared juices and raw blended soups daily. Juice fasting is a good way to accomplish the colon cleanse, candida cleanse, parasite cleanse, kidney cleanse, and liver cleanse all at the same time.

There are different theories on the best method to complete a juice fast;

through juicing or blending fruits and vegetables. Juicing will press the juice from the fruits or vegetables, leaving only the juice and eliminating the pulp from the fruit or vegetables. This is a good method but can also become very expensive because you will yield a little juice in comparison to the amount of fruits and vegetables being used. Because juicing produces only the juice, it will be taken up into the cells quicker. Juicing may cause constipation due to the lack of fiber pushing the toxic waste through the colon. In which case, it is a good idea to perform an enema to help to eliminate the waste.

Blending the fruits and vegetables in a high-speed blender will keep the pulp and fiber within the juice; also known as smoothies. With fiber intact, your colon will stay in the game, and you will be less constipated. The blended fruits and vegetables will retain fiber to help eliminate toxic waste, but you may still need to perform an enema on occasion.

Which method is better, juicing or blending, is dependent upon your preference. I personally like blending fruits and vegetables because it retains fiber and yields more juice, so I save money in the long run. I also make sure to perform coffee enemas to help to detoxify my liver at the same time as detoxifying my colon and other organs in my body.

If you are going to enlist only the juice fast, you can also use some psyllium husk or ground flaxseed to get your fiber to help eliminate constipation. The juicing regimen of detoxification and healing is expounded upon in more detail in chapter 9, as I personally used this method as one of the ways I healed cancer.

Water Fasting

What happens when you have tried every method of detoxification, and nothing seems to be working for you? This is when your health and detoxification need to be taken to the next level and embark upon the most extreme detox regimen of all, The Water Fast.

There are occasions when all of the previous detoxification methods will not work for various issues. The main reason is due to a systemic candida condition in the digestive tract, which is one of the most difficult conditions to rid from the body. There are also certain autoimmune conditions where the water fast is the only method that will work to re-set the body.

There was an occasion where the systemic candida within my gut had caused so many problems that none of the other detoxification methods were working any longer, when they previously worked before. I, therefore, turned to water fasting and continued coffee enemas to cleanse the liver of increased toxins being released through fasting.

One of the benefits of water fasting is that it gives your digestive tract a much-needed rest, so it is able to repair itself. The digestive tract normally takes 14 days to heal completely, so if you have extreme intestinal permeability issues, this can help you to heal.

What I noticed through water fasting is that if you have systemic candida in the digestive tract, you will notice that your tongue becomes white as the candida is leaving the body, increased body odors, pasty mouth, bad breath, acne, rashes, and boils will come out, and many of the other healing crisis symptoms discussed in the next section.

Water fasting is biblical and has been done for thousands of years. Although, water fasting should be monitored closely by a qualified physician to monitor blood pressure, heart rate, and pulse. There are even specific water fasting retreats where you can complete a water fasting program safely and be monitored the entire time. For those who want to go to a retreat for water fasting, I suggest Tanglewood Wellness Center, run by Loren Lockwood and located in Costa Rica. Please tell Loren that you read it in my book. The website is http://www.tanglewoodwellnesscenter.com.

I do not suggest starting off with the water fast because it is so extreme and needs to be monitored. However, when all other avenues of detoxification have been exhausted unsuccessfully, water fasting may be an option for you. Please discuss this with your qualified naturopathic doctor or go to the water fasting retreat listed above. Water fasting should not be done by those with advanced cancer as the body needs all the energy to heal and fasting with late-stage cancer can send the body into advanced adrenal fatigue. Fasting can put too much stress on a body which is already in extreme stress with cancer, so please see a qualified physician when undertaking fasting.

Detoxification Symptoms & The Healing Crisis

While detoxing the body, you will most likely experience flu like symptoms that can last a few days or more. This is a sign that your body is ridding itself of toxins. Any ailments you have had in the past will come out in reverse order of when you first experienced them. Here are some other die-off symptoms you may experience. These symptoms tell you that detoxification is working.

- Headache, fatigue, dizziness, nausea, diarrhea, bloating, gas, constipation, excess gas, and burping.
- Increased joint or muscle pain, swollen glands, elevated heart rate, sweating, and fever.
- Chills, cold feeling in your extremities, recurring vaginal, prostate, and sinus infections.
- Body itchiness, hives, skin breakouts, acne, boils, or rashes.

If the "healing crisis" is too severe, you may want to slow down a bit, so as not to release too many toxins at once. To slow down or to release the toxins quicker, drink more water, dry heat saunas, infrared saunas, exercise, rest, and take 2,000 mg of vitamin C daily (if not on the Budwig protocol).

By conducting these cleanses, you will be able to free yourself from the many ailments that may have plagued you for years. Keep on a regular plan to detoxify your body at least annually. Those with cancer should detox twice a year. I like to detox as the New Year begins, but it can be done at any time you feel sluggish or need a boost.

All of the methods of detoxifying the body will help you to rid your body of toxins, try the different ones and see which ones work best for you. Do not perform them all at the same time or you could detoxify your body too fast, which will cause further problems. Go slow, relax, and know that you are doing a great thing for your body and helping to prevent disease or rid your body of disease.

When detoxing from cancer, especially advanced cancer, you may experience what is known as Lysing symptoms. In layman's terms, Lysing is just the breaking down of the cancer cell, which releases additional potassium, uric acid, and phosphorous into the blood. Lysing also depletes calcium reserves. If after starting any alternative treatments, you experience extreme headaches, vomiting, diarrhea, muscle cramps, lethargy, or confusion, this means that the toxins from cancer are being released too quickly. Coffee enemas can help to alleviate pain and get rid of the toxins in the system. Liquid Bentonite clay also helps to bind toxins and move them out of the body.

Lysing symptoms that go on for an extended period of time can lead to kidney failure, cardiovascular issues, seizures, and other organ damage. It is important that if you experience lysing, to spread out your alternative treatments, utilize coffee enemas, and liquid Bentonite clay to alleviate the toxic load on the body.

Now that you know how to detoxify the body, you can move onto what to feed the body to reverse cancer and other diseases naturally. In the following Chapters, I will be discussing the protocols I used to heal cancer naturally. During these protocols, I was doing the detoxification regimen at the same time.

Chapter 7
The Power of Enzymes

As previously discussed, cancer is caused from an overabundance of toxins in the body, a deficiency in vital nutrients, and an acidic condition in the body. Cancer happens with a change in the cell; "The process of cell change, in which, a cell loses its ability to control its rate of division, and thus becomes a tumor cell, is called cell transformation." It has also been proven by Dr. Otto Warburg, in 1931, that the Cancer cell needs an anaerobic environment; meaning without oxygen, to thrive and that cancer cells die in the presence of an aerobic condition, or infusion of oxygen.

Where the power of enzymes comes into play is with the breaking down of protein, carbohydrates, and fats. However, we are mostly concerned with breaking down the protein barrier of the cancer cell wall, so this is where enzymes are beneficial in fighting cancer.

Enzymes

Your pancreas, when working normally, makes enough enzymes to break down the foods you eat. The term Proteolytic enzymes refer to the substances that aid in the breakdown and assimilation of proteins within the body. The various enzymes within the pancreas help to digest foods. Lipases help to digest fats, proteases help to digest proteins, and amylases help to digest carbohydrates. We are most concerned with the proteases and breaking down the protein layer of the cancer cell.

A cancer cell contains a protein layer that surrounds the cell and needs to be broken through to get to the malignant cell within. There are two fruits that contain this pancreatic enzyme that breaks down protein; one is the Hawaiian papaya; called Papain, which are mostly genetically modified organisms (GMO), and the other is pineapple; known as Bromelain.

The protein layer of the cancer cell needs to be penetrated in order to deliver oxygen into the cancer cell thus reversing the cancer. In order to get the oxygenated mixture of the Budwig Protocol; which I will discuss in the next chapter, or any of the other alternative cancer treatments to the center of the cancer cell, you first need to open up the protein layer covering the cancer wall with a pancreatic enzyme known as Bromelain or Papain; which is found in pineapple or papaya. Opening up the protein layer covering the cancer cell wall will enable the alternative treatment to reach the center of the cell and the cancer itself.

The pineapple or papaya is a key ingredient because it is a protein digesting enzyme, which breaks down the protein barrier to the cancer cell wall. Anything you ingest after eating the pineapple or papaya will make its way directly into the cancer cell. So, you must be very aware of what you eat or drink after ingesting pineapple or papaya. You may not have any sugar, caffeine, processed foods, or various meat products while on this plan, as it will interfere with your healing and may bring on worse conditions. It is a scientific fact that cancer feeds on sugar and when you ingest sugar, the cancer will grow and multiply very rapidly and exponentially. Consider when you go to get a PET scan and you are given a mixture of glucose to drink, the cancer cells go straight for the glucose mixture, which lights up the PET scan like a Christmas tree, making it easy to detect the cancer cells.

Sugar also suppresses the immune system for hours after ingesting it. If your immune system is already suppressed due to cancer, you cannot fight off cancer and the cancer will continue to multiply. When I had cancer, I had tested out this theory multiple times, by eating sugar, and the end result was that I could literally feel my body shutting down, the immune system crashing, the lethargy was immediate, and I would have to go to sleep for 3 to 4 hours in order to recover. This is no joke, do not eat sugar when you have cancer, to do so is signing your death warrant. So, if you don't want your cancer to spread and grow, you definitely need to stay away from sugar.

Another forbidden chemical to stay away from if you have cancer, is Caffeine. Caffeine is also highly acidic on the body and carries low oxygen to the cells, which also helps cancer to multiply. Unfortunately, the morning cup of Joe will have to go, but coffee enemas can stay, as coffee enemas do not have the same effect on the body as drinking the coffee.

Beef, Chicken, and Fish are also forbidden for a time, while trying to heal cancer because they contain protein. What happens is that when you eat meat, the pancreatic enzymes within your body go to work to try to break down your meal and the meat takes a lot of pancreatic enzymes. So, if the enzymes are busy working on breaking down the heavy protein meal you just ate, then they aren't available to break down the cancer cell wall. Let the enzymes do their work on the protein coating found on the outside of the cancer cell wall and not on the meat ingested. This means that meat is high in protein and will take the pancreatic enzymes away from the cancer cell in order to digest the meat. You don't want any interference of your digestive enzymes, they need to specifically work on the protein membrane of the cancer cell wall, so you can effectively get the oxygen to the center of the cancer cell and start reversing cancer naturally.

The idea of using pancreatic enzymes to assist in healing cancer came in the 1960s from Dr. William Donald Kelley, a dentist who healed his own pancreatic, liver, and intestinal cancer naturally. His therapy, "Metabolic therapy," tailors the therapy to each individual based upon their metabolic type. After Dr. Kelley had healed his own terminal cancer, he went on to assist 33,000 others, over a 30-year period, to successfully treat their own cancers. Of course, he was attacked by the government, had his dental license suspended, and his therapy was kept from mainstream medicine.

Due to the success of Dr. Kelley's Metabolic therapy and using pancreatic enzymes to assist in healing cancer, this is where I had come up with the idea of utilizing the enzymes in their natural form. Since I didn't have money to afford the pancreatic enzyme supplements, I researched the natural form of pancreatic enzymes and found the Bromelain and Papain. Using pineapple, as the enzyme, was not only more cost effective, but made more sense because it comes directly from God's pharmacy.

While I was healing cancer, I used to cut up a fresh pineapple weekly and then eat a few bites of pineapple at a time before utilizing the other healing cancer protocols. Eating the pineapple helped to open up my cancer cell, so the other alternative methods could get directly into the cell and reverse the cancer naturally.

I would also utilize imagery as a positive reinforcement to battling cancer, so while I was eating the pineapple, I was imagining that my cancer cell was opening and was going to receive the oxygen boost from all of the alternative treatments. The mind is a powerful tool, in addition to proper nutrition, to use in healing the body. After eating the pineapple, I used The Budwig protocol, fresh vegetable juices, and apricot kernels to deliver the fatal blow to the cancer itself, all of which will be explained in the following chapters.

Chapter 8
The Budwig Protocol

After I had figured out that I had cancer, I was unemployed, and had just completed grad school, I could now pay attention to healing myself naturally. While I was sitting in front of the computer, I was crying and prayed to the Lord to help me heal myself of cancer. This is when I was led to the Budwig Protocol, in all of its glory, and it was the first protocol that I came upon. Not only was I impressed with the science behind the Budwig Protocol but was also swayed by the fact that it was so inexpensive, non-invasive, and easy to administer.

Dr. Johanna Budwig: a resident of Germany, had a doctorate in Physics, Biochemistry and was also a licensed Pharmacist. She had also gone back to school and became a holistic practitioner. Dr. Budwig had worked as a senior expert for pharmaceuticals and fats at the Federal Institute for Fats Research in Germany. She had written various books and scientific papers on cancer and the role of fats and was nominated for the Nobel Prize seven times. Dr. Budwig had successfully treated over 2,400 people with cancer and other diseases in the 50 years she was practicing.

Dr. Budwig had discovered that cancer was a symptom caused by the deficiency of good fats within the cells. She began with the basic discovery of Dr. Otto Warburg, who years earlier won the Nobel Prize for his discovery that cancer cannot live in an oxygenated environment, and then she expanded upon the idea by discovering how to get oxygen directly into the cancer cell.

According to Dr. Budwig, combining flax oil and low-fat cottage cheese results in creating a sulphurated protein, which infuses the cancer cell with oxygen, thereby reversing the nutrient deficiency and reversing the cancer naturally. Dr. Johanna Budwig had over 90% cancer reversal rate by utilizing her discovery.

Dr. Budwig had noticed that most typical cancer patients had a greenish-yellowish substance in their blood, and they were lacking in the Omega 3 essential fatty acids that were present with most healthy patients. Dr. Budwig had concluded that the lack of good fats was the reason why patients became so weak and anemic.

In order to reverse cancer, Dr. Budwig had infused the body with good fats, thereby reversing cancer and other diseases. The issue is to reverse the root cause of cancer, not the symptom of cancer. The symptom of cancer is the tumor, but the root cause has to do with a nutritional deficiency and fungus, in most cases. It makes complete sense that if you have fungus and/or parasites growing within your cells you will not be able to get the sufficient nutrients you need, thereby creating a nutritional deficiency. Therefore, getting to the root cause and healing what causes cancer in the first place, will help to alleviate the symptoms of cancer.

In many instances, Dr. Budwig had begun treating patients using her protocol, when some of the patients were on their death bed with only a few weeks or days to live. These terminal patients were sent home to die by their traditional doctors after the traditional medicine failed to heal them. Many of these patients could not eat and had to be given the flax oil as an enema to start. By using the flax oil as an enema, the benefits were passed through the colon walls, and the patients began to heal. Once the body began to utilize the benefits of the flax oil through the colon walls, the patients began to heal to the point where they could now eat and ingest the Budwig protocol orally. Many of her patients were healed of cancer, along with other serious diseases, by utilizing her protocol.

Due to the success rate of the Budwig protocol and the many conferences she held, Dr. Johanna Budwig was taken to court by the Central Committee for Cancer Research based upon her statements about healing cancer. Due to the numerous conclusive papers and documents that Dr. Budwig possessed, regarding the efficacy of her treatment of cancer, the judge pulled aside the Central Committee for Cancer Research and told them not to push this matter any further as it would create a scandal in the entire scientific community. Dr. Budwig had so much proof of healing cancer patients using her protocol, after they were sent home to die by traditional doctors, that to pursue it further would have been a blow to the entire medical industry.

The Budwig protocol is also said to heal various cancers and diseases; such as, throat cancer, breast cancer, colon cancer, liver cancer, kidney cancer, lung cancer, leukemia, skin cancer, melanoma, pancreatic cancer, bladder cancer, cervical cancer, prostate cancer, rectal cancer, testicular cancer, esophageal cancer, bone cancer, appendix cancer, stomach cancer, anal cancer, heart infarction, brain tumors, autoimmune diseases, AIDS, asthma, fibromyalgia, diabetes, eczema, multiple sclerosis, acne, psoriasis, blood pressure, heart disease, and arthritic conditions. This protocol will also work for cancer in cats or dogs.

How it Works

The Budwig Protocol consists of a mixture of low-fat organic cottage cheese and flaxseed oil. According to Johanna Budwig, the blending of the low-fat cottage cheese and flax oil provides a sulphurated protein that becomes water soluble and is able to easily absorb through the cancer cell wall. When the mixture penetrates the cancer cell wall, it creates a torrent of oxygen to the cancer cell and reverses cancer naturally. When the two are combined, they are able to heal cancer within the body by bringing oxygenated protein into the cancer cell. This process helps to correct the Omega 3 deficiency within the cells and reverses cancer naturally.

The oxygen infusion into the cancer cells is caused by the electrons from the seed oils in the mixture, which will come to the surface of the body and react to the photons from the sun. This is the reason why it is imperative to get at least 15 minutes of sunlight daily after consuming the Budwig Protocol; it will aid the interaction of electron rich foods in order to reverse cancer naturally.

Make sure that you use an organic; cold pressed, refrigerated Flax Oil with no additives. You should also be using a low-fat organic cottage cheese that does not contain any milk from cows treated with the bovine growth hormone; Rbst or Rbgh. If you cannot handle milk products efficiently, you may use kefir although I am not sure how effective this is as a treatment method. The mixture of cottage cheese and flax oil changes its chemical composition when it is emulsified together, so those people who are lactose intolerant or have dairy allergies, have not shown any aversion to the Budwig protocol.

The Recipe

The mixture of cottage cheese and flax oil needs to be two to one. This means that if you use two tablespoons of cottage cheese, you need one tablespoon of flax oil. You will need an immersion hand-held stick type blender, in order to make this properly, which you can pick up fairly inexpensively at a Wal-Mart or Target type store. I put four tablespoons of organic cottage cheese (needs to be from cows not treated with the Rbst or Rbgh hormones) to two tablespoons of Flax Oil together with a small amount of unsweetened almond milk. Emulsify the mixture before adding anything else to the combination. When it is blended together it should resemble the consistency of custard or thick yogurt. You must make sure that there is no separation of the flax oil from the cottage cheese, or the mixture will not become water soluble to penetrate the cancer cell. These two ingredients need to be bonded together to be effective.

After the mixture is emulsified, you can get a bit creative. I have added more unsweetened almond milk, blueberries, ground flaxseed, and a banana to make a drinkable shake. Do not mix pineapple with this mixture, as it will tend to turn the mixture bitter and coagulate. In my opinion, making a drinkable shake out of the Budwig mixture is a great way to take it because you can drink it down fast. Do not let the mixture sit around as flax oil and flax seed goes rancid quickly.

The Budwig protocol also tastes good as a thick yogurt, with a few additions mixed in to make it more palatable. The method in which Dr. Budwig used her protocol was to add 1-2 Tablespoons of freshly ground flax seeds to the bottom of a bowl. Then put a layer of fruit or nuts on top of the ground flaxseed. Top the fruit or nuts with the freshly blended base mixture of the flaxseed oil and cottage cheese and you can add a bit of raw honey to sweeten it up. You can use any type of fruit; bananas, berries, cherries, apples, peaches, to add to the mixture. You can use raw walnuts, raw almonds, and raw brazil nuts to the mixture as well. When you mix all of this together, you have a tasty mixture that is very filling for breakfast or anytime of the day.

Adding ground flax seeds will also help to heal cancer because you are adding more Omega 3's into your body and flax seeds also contain amygdalin (more on this in a later chapter), which is also known to kill cancer. Make sure that any flax seeds you buy are in whole form and fresh, they need to be ground up daily and will go rancid within 15 minutes of grinding and lose their efficacy. Buying ground flax seeds in the stores is a waste of money because they are already rancid. Buy them whole, keep them in the freezer, and grind them yourself daily using a coffee grinder.

As with most alternative methods for cancer, there are treatments that are compatible with protocols and ones that aren't compatible. This is where many people make mistakes with healing cancer naturally because they end up doing too many various alternative treatments at once, not realizing that their treatments are not compatible with one another and can cause further damage or even death.

Many people have stated that the Budwig protocol didn't work for them, when in fact; the issue was not with the Budwig protocol, but the fact that the person was utilizing incompatible treatments, which will lessen the efficacy of the Budwig protocol.

Treatments Compatible with Budwig

Certain treatments are compatible with the Budwig Protocol and can be utilized, such as meditation, laughter, prayer, positive outlook, healing affirmations, exercise, detoxification, sunlight, infrared sauna, dry heat saunas, juicing vegetables, amygdalin (aka; laetrile or natural vitamin B17), and enzyme therapy.

Supplements, teas, and juices you may take are milk thistle, seaweed, aloe vera, spirulina, wheatgrass juice, Essiac formula, and chlorella. You can also drink specific caffeine free teas, such as peppermint, Pau D'arco, Valerian root, green tea, and other herbal teas without additives or sugar. You can use all the spices to spice your food.

The Budwig Protocol should be continued for five years or as a general maintenance program for life. After five years, you can gradually loosen your dietary habits, but not too extreme as before cancer.

Treatments NOT Compatible with Budwig

Do not take hormones, birth control pills, cortisone, painkillers, chemotherapy, radiation, narcotics, food preservatives, GMOs, alcohol, sugar, caffeine, aspirin, medications, ozone, high oxygen treatments, cesium chloride, hydrogen peroxide therapy or injections, fluoride, aspartame, tap water, alkaline water, pesticides, chlorine, the wrong fats, butter, margarine, hormone laden meats, factory farmed fish, pastries, processed foods, anti-oxidants, IP-6, Protandim, Protocel, vitamin C, vitamin E, selenium, and stress.

To take any of the incompatible treatments along with the Budwig Protocol will interfere with the positive effects of the protocol and can even be fatal. It has been said that when someone abandons the Budwig protocol too early and returns to their old dietary habits that cancer will come back, and it will not be able to be healed again, even if going back to the vegetarian diet and Budwig Protocol. Johanna Budwig had stated that if this happens that there will be a quick demise within a couple of weeks.

I have personally done this, and I was on my deathbed within weeks, this is NOT a joke. When I abandoned the Budwig protocol in April of 2010, after only 11 months of taking it, I had gone back to taking the birth control pill and eating donuts daily. Within 6 months, cancer was back and so I started back on the Budwig protocol, while still on birth control pills and eating sugar daily. By Christmas of 2010, I was sleeping 21 hours per day, back in the "brain fog," and felt my body shutting down.

The only reason I am here to write about the fatal dangers of stopping and re-starting the Budwig Protocol is by a divine miracle from the grace of God. When I was lying on my couch and I felt as if I were dying, I was crying out to the Lord. At that point, I was so tired of fighting cancer and detoxing that I had had enough. I basically told God that "I was done detoxing and that if he wanted to heal me from cancer that he would have to do it himself." After going to bed for the night, I awoke the next morning with an extreme urgency to go to the toilet. I ran to the bathroom with extreme diarrhea four times that morning. After the third time, of my urgent visits, to the bathroom, I had felt the "brain fog" lift off of me like a shade being pulled up from a window. It was the most amazing feeling because at that moment, I felt as if I was healed, and I was feeling more energy again and more like myself. I feel God gave me a second chance at life to be able to bring this important information to the public and let people know that God had already created all of the tools to heal disease and cancer naturally, it just takes time to find the proper alternative method.

The reason that I tell you about this fatal mistake that I made is, that you won't make the same mistake. Why will you rarely see this important information, of starting and stopping Budwig, in many other books written about alternative treatments for cancer? Most books that contain information about the Budwig protocol are written by people who have never had cancer personally and therefore have never used these treatments on themselves in a cancerous environment. Other books either fail to mention or barely mention this very important fact; to ignore this is definitely fatal!

Another reason why you may not have heard this before is because any patient who has abandoned the protocol or combined incompatible therapies with the Budwig protocol is no longer alive to talk about how dangerous it is, if used incorrectly. Not only have I done it but have seen countless people tell me that the Budwig protocol didn't work for them, and when I question them as to how they were using it, every single person had been combining it incorrectly or using it with incompatible therapies. I had also known of people who had died because they incorrectly combined the wrong foods, supplements, or treatments with the Budwig Protocol.

This protocol is so effective that advanced cancer patients need to be aware of the lysing symptoms, which I discussed in the detoxification chapter, and be diligent about using coffee enemas and other detoxification methods to rid the body of the toxins from lysing. When starting this protocol, the cancer will begin to dissipate, causing all of the toxins to be released in the body. If you don't use coffee enemas to rid the body of toxic poisons, you can die due to the overabundance of toxins.

The lysing symptoms happened to me many times and did cause issues. Within the first few months of starting Budwig and all of the other alternative treatments, I experienced profuse sweating, chills, fever, vomiting, and diarrhea. Once I spread out all of my alternative therapies throughout the day and continued to detox my body, the lysing symptoms stopped.

The Budwig protocol MUST be followed for at least five years, although it would be beneficial to maintain a daily regimen of the mixture for the rest of your life. You cannot abandon the program when you feel that you are well enough and resume eating or drinking what you did before because the cancer will come back at full force and no amount of diet changing at that point will matter and people have been said to die within weeks.

Another cautionary note regarding ingesting flaxseed oil; also known as linseed oil, is from a study conducted in France by The National Institute of Alimentary Research. The study included injecting pregnant rats with 100 grams of linseed oil, which caused the death of all the young either at birth or two weeks later. According to William Fischer in response to the research results, "Although the amount of linseed oil fed the female rats in this study was proportionately much greater than would normally be ingested by a pregnant woman supplementing her diet with this nutrient, the results of this important research certainly indicate that a woman who is (or suspects she might be) pregnant should not include linseed oil in her diet until after giving birth and weaning the child."

Before you decide to enlist the Budwig Protocol as a part of your healing, make sure that you are ready to make the commitment to continue the program for at least five years. This protocol can be incorporated daily for the rest of your life as a way to supplement the "good fats" that are deficient in your body. Although, be very careful that when you begin the Budwig Protocol that you can no longer go back to the old lifestyle and eating habits that gave you cancer in the first place.

I don't mean to frighten anyone by the extreme warnings to the Budwig protocol because this is the most effective therapy for cancer I have researched and experimented with. This is a complete lifestyle change, and in my opinion, is a much better alternative than that of chemotherapy, radiation, and surgery. This is a decision that you need to make on your own as to what form of healing you want to take. You will find many compatible recipes, for the Budwig Protocol, in a later chapter, which will make it easier for you to transition to this lifestyle change.

After enlisting the Budwig protocol for cancer, I added another compatible facet of alternative healing to my daily regimen. The reason for combining the various therapies that I did was to combat cancer from every direction in a safe way. In the next chapter, I will discuss the importance of juicing and its beneficial effect upon cancer.

Chapter 9

Drink Your Vegetables

Every morning, after I had taken the Budwig protocol; I had started making my green juice for consumption. As was stated by Dr. Norman Walker; "Vegetable juices are the builders and regenerators of the body, they contain all the amino acids, minerals, salts, enzymes, and vitamins needed by the human body provided that they are used fresh, raw, and without preservatives and that they have been properly extracted from the vegetables."

Juicing is where the juice from a vegetable or fruit is extracted from the pulp, leaving only the juice. A masticating type of juicer or blender will blend the entire vegetable or fruit, leaving the pulp within the juice (smoothie). Different types of juicers available on the market are Omega, Champion, Jack LaLane, Hurom, Breville juice fountain, and many others. Different types of Masticating Blenders on the market are the; Vitamix, Blendtec, and Montel Williams. It is based upon personal preference as to which one will work best for you, which I briefly touched upon in the detoxification chapter.

The Benefits of Vegetable Juices

The benefits of vegetable juices are that the juice can assimilate into the body quicker because there is no fiber to digest. With juicing, you are giving your digestive system a much-needed rest to heal and repair itself, while still getting all of the vitamins, enzymes, and minerals you need within the juice. This is a definite benefit to juicing over blending. However, juicing can be very costly because you have to use a large amount of vegetables to get a small amount of juice. I like juicing, but I could not afford it while I was healing cancer naturally, so I opted for vegetable smoothies instead.

The Benefits of Vegetable Smoothies

A vegetable smoothie is a combination of vegetables blended with a high-powered blender, strong enough to pulverize anything that goes into it, called a masticating blender. The benefit of a vegetable smoothie, as opposed to green juice, is that a smoothie leaves the pulp within the juice and is therefore a great method of detoxification and can also be used for a juice feast. As talked about in the detoxification chapter, this is a great way to detoxify the colon and other organs in the body.

For those with advanced cancers, I have noticed that most people will have intestinal permeability issues due to the toxins, chemotherapy, radiation, or antibiotics which have altered their gut flora. It may be too difficult for those with advanced cancers to digest the pulp from the vegetables. Therefore, it may be necessary to use a juicer first to help to replace the lost minerals within the body, without the added strain of trying to digest the fibers from the vegetables. Again, which works best for you is a personal opinion. Try both and see which one works for you.

Gerson Therapy

Dr. Max Gerson, a medical doctor from Germany, had begun using metabolic therapy to heal many "incurable" diseases. Although he had first set up a medical practice in 1919 in Germany, he had immigrated to the United States in 1936 to set up his medical practice in New York. Dr. Gerson's therapy utilized many vegetable juices throughout the day, supplements, and coffee enemas. It is with his therapy of drinking vegetable juices and coffee enemas that so many patients have healed from cancer utilizing this method.

Dr. Gerson, like many other doctors who heal cancer naturally, was referred to as a quack by the medical establishment. And even though he had written books and published over 50 papers regarding his findings, the American Medical Association and the National Cancer Institute refused to look at his successful treatment for cancer and other diseases. He eventually lost his license to practice medicine in the state of New York and moved his practice to California, where it still sits today.

The Gerson Institute, located in San Diego, CA. with a clinic in Tijuana, Mexico and also one in Budapest, Hungary, was founded by Charlotte Gerson, Dr. Max Gerson's daughter. Charlotte Gerson passed away peacefully at the age of 96 in 2019. The Gerson Institute is still operational and is run by qualified doctors trained in the Gerson method. The Gerson Institute practices successful treatment for cancer and other diseases and people from all over the world flock to the Gerson center for treatment.

The Gerson treatment utilizes 13 fresh juices daily, from only organically grown fruits and vegetables. Five coffee enemas per day are used to help cleanse the liver of toxins. The patients are also put on a strict diet with no salt, no sugar, and very little meat. The Gerson method also utilizes supplements within their therapy.

While I was healing cancer naturally, I only utilized portions of the Gerson method due to the high cost of the supplements. I only juiced 3 times per day and maintained a very strict diet. I did not start utilizing coffee enemas until the second time I had cancer, but I was detoxifying my body and was using Dr. Hulda Clark's method of detoxifying the liver. Some of the supplements used in Gerson therapy are incompatible with the Budwig protocol, so that is another reason why I didn't utilize the supplemental therapy.

Which Vegetables to Use

Your personal health challenges will determine which fruits or vegetables are best to use. If you have cancer, you will want to stay away from too many fruits that are high in sugar content because cancer feeds on sugar. So, it would be best to stick with vegetables that are low in sugar. It is always best to juice raw vegetables and fruits separately and not mix the two, but it is understandable that when you are new to juicing you may need to add a slice of apple for taste. It is also imperative to rotate the fruits and vegetables, so you are not overloading on one specific vegetable or fruit.

The basics of most juicing recipes, and some of my favorites include spinach, kale, celery, cucumber, carrots, apples, parsley, romaine, red bell pepper and beets. You can start with these to begin with and then experiment with other fruits and vegetables. Some of the juice recipes I had used can be found in the recipe section of this book.

Help, I've Turned Orange

Juicing carrots are very beneficial for cancer due to the beta carotene properties, which carry a live electrical charge, and are cleansing the liver. According to Dr. Norman Walker, "Raw carrot juice is a natural solvent for ulcerous and cancerous conditions." Mostly all cancer patients have a clogged liver and when you juice carrots, it will cleanse the liver and sometimes will discolor your skin a yellowish/orange tint. The reason that carrots have this effect is not due to the beta carotene in the carrot, but that the liver is clogged and is getting a much-needed cleansing. So, be thankful if you turn orange as this means that your body is cleansing itself. The orange/yellow tint will dissipate eventually.

Goitrogenic Foods

Those people who are diagnosed with hypothyroidism or low thyroid should not juice certain raw fruits and vegetables in copious amounts because it will negatively affect the thyroid causing extreme weight gain. If you currently have low thyroid or hypothyroid, please use the goitrogenic fruits or vegetables on a rotation and sparingly. If you do not have a thyroid issue, then you can safely juice raw vegetables and fruits.

You can still juice or make smoothies in its raw state, or you can also steam the vegetables first to remove the goitrogenic properties and then also drink the juice that the vegetables were steamed in, so you don't lose the vitamin and mineral content. I usually add the steamed juice directly into my Vitamix to make my green smoothies or raw soups. I also still juice raw vegetables but now rotate the goitrogens.

The reason that I had learned about goitrogens was because I had a negative reaction from juicing too many goitrogenic greens at once. By January of 2011, after my second bout with cancer in December of 2010 and God saving me from certain death, I had enough energy back to start juicing again and was juicing around 100 ounces per day of spinach and kale. I couldn't figure out why I kept gaining 10 lbs. per month, when I was on a juice fast and hiking 50 miles per week.

I was later diagnosed with low thyroid and advanced adrenal fatigue, after I had already gained 50 lbs. from juicing. Although, it was a no-brainer, as I could tell that I already had a thyroid condition from the extreme symptoms I had experienced, and the diagnosis just confirmed what I already knew. One of my downfalls is that I do not know the word, Moderation. With me, it is all or nothing and juicing that much spinach and kale, without rotating my vegetables, had caused extreme weight gain. There is nothing more horrible than gaining weight from vegetables because everyone assumes that I must sit around eating fattening foods, when in fact, my diet was better than most.

My advice to you is to please rotate your vegetables and don't go overboard with any one vegetable but use moderation. The following is a list of goitrogenic foods that should be used sparingly and rotated often, especially if you have a thyroid condition:

Goitrogenic Foods

Kale	Spinach	Collard greens	Broccoli
Brussel sprouts	Alfalfa sprouts	Cauliflower	Cabbage
Kohlrabi	Mustard greens	Radishes	Soy
Rutabagas	Soy milk	Mustard	Tempeh
Tofu	Soybean oil	Soy lecithin	Anything with soy
Turnips	Bamboo shoots	Millet	Peanuts
Pears	Pine nuts	Peaches	Strawberries
Sweet potatoes	Canola	Canola oil	

Chapter 10
Apricot Kernels

When I first began eating apricot kernels, as part of my cancer therapy, I would ask God why he would make it so difficult to reach the beneficial life-giving seed in the middle of the apricot. I am guessing that God wants to see just how badly you want to live. In Genesis 1:29, the Lord says, "I give you every seed-bearing plant on the face of the whole earth and every tree that has fruit with seed in it. They will be yours for food."

Dr. Ernest T. Krebs Jr. had discovered that on the inside of an apricot is a hard-shelled pit about the size of a marble. It is within this hard shell that offers a miracle. When the pit is cracked open it reveals a small kernel that is pure amygdalin, also known as vitamin B17. Amygdalin contains a cyanide compound that is not toxic to the body but is toxic to a cancer cell. Unlike a normal cell, the cancer cell contains a special enzyme that allows the cyanide to be released in the amygdalin. So, the cyanide only targets cancer cells but leaves the normal cells alone.

Amygdalin is found in many foods that you eat daily, such as, apple seeds, apricot kernels, bitter almonds, wheatgrass, millet, barley, lima beans, lentils, corn, strawberries, blackberries, raspberries, loganberries, boysenberries, cranberries, elderberries, mulberries, gooseberries, huckleberries, sweet potatoes, flaxseed, flaxseed oil, kidney beans, cassava, cherries, peaches, plums, and prunes. Although, the highest concentration of amygdalin is found in the apricot kernel.

Many people mistakenly interchange the terms amygdalin, laetrile, and vitamin B17 to mean the same thing. Amygdalin, also known as vitamin B17, is the natural form. Laetrile is the compound derived from amygdalin. According to William Fischer "The name Laetrile, referring to an apricot-pit formula, developed at the John Beard Memorial Foundation in San Francisco is a registered trademark coined in 1952 by its discoverer, Ernst Krebs Jr. Laetrile is a combination of the term levorotary (having the ability to turn polarized light to the left) and nitrile (an organic compound in which nitrogen exists with all three of the displaced hydrogen atoms)." "Laetrile is two molecules of glucose, one molecule of benzaldehyde and one molecule of hydrogen cyanide (HCN)." Laetrile is a more concentrated version derived from amygdalin and used as IV therapy or in supplemental form.

As I was conducting my research, I found many claims of people being healed from cancer through eating the apricot kernels daily. There are also reports of various populations of people who do not get cancer because their diet contains foods high in amygdalin. Once those people adopt a western diet, they also succumb to cancer.

There is a tribe of people in Pakistan; known as the Hunza tribe, who live on the base of the Himalayan Mountains. These people are known as the Hunzakuts, and they have been studied because they have never had one incident of cancer. When they were studied, it was found that their eating habits varied greatly from the traditional western diet. The Hunzakuts ate grain, meats, milk, and fruit. They had a massive amount of apricot trees and ate apricots during the summer months and then dried the apricots for the winter months.

The Hunza tribe also used apricot kernels for eating and to press into oil. One item that stood out from all other diets, is that the Hunzakuts ate about 30-50 apricot seeds daily as part of their usual diet. According to Dr. Ernest Krebs Jr., this high concentration of B17 was found to prevent cancer from forming and in larger doses it was found to heal cancer in someone that already had the disease.

Eating seeds is an innate response in the wild animal population of gorillas, bears, and other animals. It has been observed that animals that are given apricots to eat will often tear away the fleshy part of the fruit to get to the pit on the inside, break open the shell with their teeth, and eat the kernel on the inside. Animals have also been observed cracking the seeds open by hitting them against a rock or hard object. Animals that are held in captivity, as in zoos, without being given a diet of apricot kernels, begin to get cancer. The point is that animals have an innate sense to realize that these seeds are beneficial to a healthy life, which is why they eat them.

In the 1970's, the Federal Drug Administration (FDA) banned all sales of vitamin B-17, stating that it is dangerous, and people could get cyanide poisoning. In my opinion, the banning of B-17 was to curtail a person from healing themselves through anything that doesn't involve a doctor or expensive, toxic pharmaceuticals. This of course is only my opinion, which is generally protected by the United States Constitution under the First Amendment right of Freedom of Speech. However, apricots and the seeds within them are still being sold in supermarkets and the FDA hasn't banned the consumption of apricots or growing your own apricot tree, as of yet.

Due to the ban on the sale of Laetrile within the United States, many alternative health clinics have opened in Mexico. In Mexico, it is legal to practice laetrile therapy and thousands of people, including past U.S. Presidents and celebrities, have been treated in cancer clinics over the border which offers IV laetrile therapy.

Aside from Laetrile IV therapy, you can also just eat the apricot kernel, which is what I did. There are sources on the internet that only sell apricot pits or apricot kernels, but they are not allowed to make claims to healing cancer, or they will be shut down by the United States government.

It is imperative that these seeds be cracked open and eaten fresh because they begin to lose their efficacy after being opened. Therefore, to get the highest concentration of B17, you must crack open the seeds daily. It is easier to crack open the seeds when you put them in a re-closeable plastic bag and hit them with a hammer to reveal the kernel on the inside. After cracking open the apricot pit to reveal the kernel inside, you must separate the hard shells from the soft kernels.

Another reason to crack open the kernels fresh is due to a fungus type mold, called an aflatoxin, that can grow on kernels that have been opened and not dried immediately. Any moisture on the kernels, allowed to sit, can grow this mycotoxin, which is carcinogenic, meaning it is known to cause cancer. Many companies online sell the apricot kernels already cracked open and vacuum packed to protect freshness. I do not know how long the kernels sit out in moisture before they are vacuum packed, so you should definitely inquire with the supplier before purchasing kernels which have already been opened.

After consuming the Budwig protocol in the morning, I would crack open the apricot seeds and grind the kernels in a coffee grinder. I would then mix the ground seeds with some organic apple sauce to make the seeds more palatable. The apricot kernels are very bitter to the taste, so I do not eat them for enjoyment, but to live. You must also be very careful with the consumption of the apricot kernels, and you should have no more than one kernel per ten pounds of body weight. So, a 150 lb. person should consume no more than 15 kernels at a time.

According to Dr. Krebs, vitamin B17 therapy should be embarked upon slowly by taking a few apricot kernels at one time and working your way up to the maximum dose. Although, you should go with a bit less because amygdalin, or vitamin B17, is also found naturally in flax seeds and many other foods, which you will be eating with the Budwig protocol. So, it is important to take vitamin B17 therapy slowly so as to not overdose on the kernels and create a healing crisis too quickly. It is also noted that vitamin B17 therapy works best when combined with pancreatic enzymes to break down the cancer cell wall prior to ingesting the apricot kernels. So, eat a bit of pineapple before consuming your apricot kernels for the maximum effect.

When your body is releasing the toxins of cancer, it will come out in many forms and can be fatal if cancer is detoxed too quickly from the body. By taking too many apricot kernels at one time, while the cancer cell is open, your body may detox too quickly from cancer and may cause nausea, vomiting, headaches, dizziness, profuse sweating, and diarrhea. This is called Lysing, which I had previously discussed in other chapters.

I had experienced lysing a few days in a row, where I ended up having increased sweats, nausea, diarrhea, and throwing up violently within 10 minutes of consuming all of the apricot kernels at one time. What I had done was open up the cancer cell wall with bromelain from the pineapple and ingested the Budwig protocol, and then I would grind the apricot seeds in a coffee grinder and eat that while my cancer cell wall was still open. I would also start mixing my green juice to detoxify my body as well. What I was doing was detoxing my body of the cancer too fast for my liver to manage all of the toxins being released and it made me violently ill. I then slowed down and did the different cancer protocols throughout the day, continued detoxification methods, along with hiking or ice skating to sweat out the toxins through my skin. By spreading out the various protocols, your body will be able to release cancer at a slower pace, which is more conducive to healing.

Chapter 11
pH Balance & Nutrition

We all know of people who are able to eat copious amounts of junk food without ever getting sick. Or those people who can smoke and drink excessive amounts of alcohol daily, but never get cancer or disease. Then there are those individuals who will end up with cancer or disease because of the foods they eat, smoking cigarettes, or excessive alcohol intake. There are also people who will get cancer or disease, even though they have never smoked or drank, and they eat healthy. All of these scenarios boil down to pH balance within the body.

In 1931, Dr. Otto Warburg had proven that oxygen kills cancer. Dr. Otto Warburg won the Nobel Prize for this discovery, but this information has been sequestered from the public unless you know where to research his findings. Diseases cannot thrive in an oxygenated environment, so the more that you increase your pH level to become more balanced on the pH scale; the more you will be able to reverse most any disease.

pH Balance refers to "potential of hydrogen" and is a measurement of whether your body is in an acidic, balanced, or alkaline state. Some people are naturally pH balanced and therefore are able to resist sickness and disease because their body naturally fights off disease. On the other hand, there are those people that are naturally acidic or the foods they eat also contribute to having an acidic body.

People that are overly acidic or overly alkaline are prone to sickness and disease. Some people need to pay extra special attention to what they eat in order to keep their body pH balanced and able to fight cancer and disease. So, how do you assess yourself to find out your pH level?

The pH scale runs from 1-14, with around 7.2 being a perfect balance. You can evaluate your pH level with pH strips that can be found in your local health food store or online. The pH strips evaluate the pH level in urine and saliva and are a fairly accurate measure of what is going on within your body. Below is an example of what a pH chart would look like.

The pH Chart

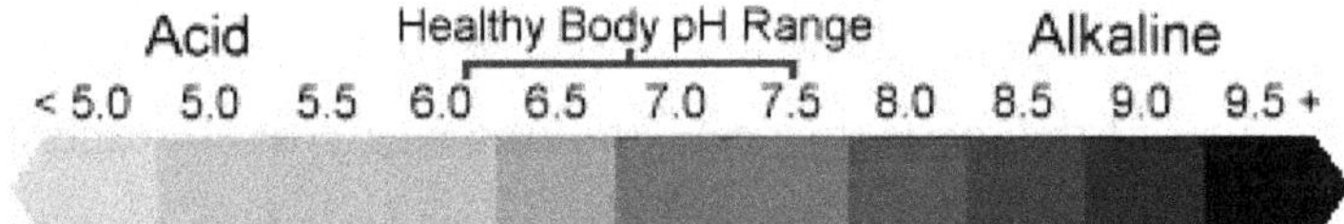

If you are sick with cancer, it is your goal to have your pH level above seven all day, every day. This is not an easy task for those of us who are naturally acidic. If you are acidic in nature, you will experience acidosis, which may create various health issues as listed in the bulleted list.

Mild acidosis can cause such problems as:

- Cardiovascular damage, constriction of blood vessels, and the reduction of oxygen.
- Bladder and kidney conditions, including kidney stones.
- Immune deficiency, Yeast/Candida overgrowth.
- Free radical damage, contributing to cancerous mutations.
- Hormone concerns, premature aging, low energy, chronic fatigue.
- Osteoporosis; weak, brittle bones, hip fractures, and bone spurs.
- Joint pain, aching muscles, and lactic acid buildup.

- Slow digestion and elimination, weight gain, obesity, and Diabetes.

Urine pH

Urine pH is extremely easy to measure, by holding the pH test strip underneath the stream of urine at any time of the day. Make sure to always use a new pH strip for each test. I personally measure my pH level, via urine, in the morning, afternoon, and evening. It gives an indication of which foods will help you to become more alkaline and which foods will make you more acidic.

Aside from really listening to how your body feels after eating certain foods, the pH test strips are a wonderful way to hammer in the principles of eating healthy foods. For instance, I would always notice that my morning urine pH would be very alkaline (around 7.5 or above) whenever I would eat raw almonds in the evening before bedtime. If I didn't eat raw almonds, my urine pH would be highly acidic at 5.0. Experiment with the alkaline food chart in this chapter to see which foods help to balance your pH level. It may be helpful to keep a food journal on which foods help to balance your pH level.

According to the Natural Health School, "Urine testing may indicate how well your body is excreting acids and assimilating minerals, especially calcium, magnesium, sodium, and potassium. These minerals function as "buffers." Buffers are substances that help maintain and balance the body against the introduction of too much acidity or too much alkalinity. Even with the proper amounts of buffers, acid or alkaline levels can become extreme. When the body ingests or produces too many of these acids or alkalis, it must excrete the excess. The urine is the perfect way for the body to remove any excess acids or alkaline substances that cannot be buffered. If the average urine pH is below 6.5 the body's buffering system is overwhelmed, a state of "autotoxication" exists, and attention should be given to lowering acid levels."

Saliva pH

Saliva pH is not as good as a predictor of what is happening within the body as it will only measure the pH level of what you last ate. I rarely ever used this method as a predictor of what was happening within my body. I had tested this method on various people who had eaten highly acidic foods, yet still tested highly alkaline through saliva pH. Urine pH is a much better predictor of pH level than saliva.

According to the Natural Health School, "The results of saliva testing may indicate the activity of digestive enzymes in the body. These enzymes are primarily manufactured by the stomach, liver, and pancreas. While saliva also utilizes buffers just like the urine, it relies on this process to a much lesser degree. If the saliva pH is too low (below 6.5), the body may be producing too many acids or may be overwhelmed by acids because it has lost the ability to adequately remove them through the urine. If the saliva pH is too high (over 6.8), the body may suffer greatly, e.g. excess gas, constipation and production of yeast, mold and fungus. Some people will have acidic pH readings from both urine and saliva—this is referred to as "double acid."

To increase pH balance within your body, you need to change your diet to include fresh vegetables. Get off of the processed foods immediately, cut out all sugars, sodas, coffee, foods that convert into sugars, genetically modified foods (GMOs), and fast foods. Only eat meals that are organic and consist of fresh fruits and vegetables. Another way to balance your pH level is by juicing green vegetables on a daily basis. Your goal is to eat a balance of foods that create a balance of acid and alkalinity in the body. This increased alkalinity increases the oxygen content within the cells which reverses cancer naturally.

If you have advanced cancer and cannot eat, I suggest making a broth from vegetables, cooking it until the vegetables become fork tender, to leech the minerals from the vegetables into the broth. Drink a few bowls of this broth daily to start to replenish the minerals in your body. Eating and drinking lots of green vegetables will start you on your path to wellness.

Dr. Emmanuel Revici had a theory regarding the pH balance of cancer patients. The theory of Dr. Revici is that people with cancer will have varying degrees of pH, which will vary dramatically from one end of the pH scale to the other end of the pH scale. Whereas someone without cancer will have a pH balance that will vary only slightly from 6.2 to a balanced state or a bit above.

A cancer patient will go from an extreme of 5.0 (highly acidic) to the other extreme of 7.5 + (highly alkaline). The more advanced your cancer is, the more the extremes will vary. I had actually experienced this many times when I tested my urine pH throughout the day, I would go from a 5.0 all the way up to an 8.0. The reason is that when cancer is releasing from the body, it sends the acidic nature of the cancer cell directly into the body, which gets released through the channels of elimination, being urine, colon, nose, throat, and skin. One can be too acidic or too alkaline and it is important to try to maintain a balanced pH level.

pH strips are fairly inexpensive and can be found at health food stores or online. If you cannot afford to get blood pH testing done, testing urine is a more accurate predictor of pH balance, than that of testing saliva. It is best to take the pH test first thing in the morning with the first morning urine and then at various times throughout the day. You will begin to notice a pattern of what you eat and how it corresponds to your pH level. Keeping this in mind with the acid/alkaline chart, it would be best to keep a food diary of which foods will help you to remain balanced all day long.

Foods You Can Eat During Cancer

Stick to 80% from the alkalizing foods and 20% from acidifying foods, although a few items of the acidifying foods are definitely NOT allowed while on the Budwig protocol or when you have cancer, so be careful when making your food choices. I noticed that many times when I eat the alkalizing foods, my urine pH test will show to be very acidic because the alkalizing foods are getting rid of the acidic content, releasing from the cancer cell, in my body. Sometimes when I would eat the acidifying foods, my urine pH would be alkaline. So, it was completely opposite of everything that most alternative health gurus tout when talking about the acid/alkaline balance.

It is also important to note that people can be too alkaline, which will also cause problems within the body. According to the late Dr. Edward Howell, being too alkaline can result when there is a lack of pancreatic enzymes present within the body to break down the protein. This is why digestive enzymes or eating pineapple are crucial to healing cancer.

One of the latest fads seems to be alkaline water, promising to increase your alkalinity and restore your health. Although, one should not go to the extreme by ingesting alkaline water because that can impair the digestive enzymes and acids within the gut, which can create further problems overall by over alkalizing the body. According to Dr. Mercola, "Alkaline water is alright to use in the short term but will create problems in long term use." Alkaline water is not compatible with the Budwig Protocol and should not be taken.

In addition to using the pH strips to test your urine for pH balance, it is important to note how you feel after eating certain foods. This is what I mean when I speak of "listening to your body." Once you are eating clean, unprocessed foods, it is easy to feel the changes in your body; you just need to pay attention. Keep a food diary to help you and write down everything you eat and how you feel after eating those types of foods. Below is the pH food chart to help you with your food choices.

ALKALIZING FOODS

VEGETABLES	FRUITS	OTHER
Garlic	Apple	Raw Apple Cider
Asparagus	Apricot	Vinegar
Fermented Veggies	Avocado	Bee Pollen
Watercress	Banana Blueberries	Lecithin Granules
Beets	Cantaloupe	Probiotic Cultures
Broccoli	Cherries	Green Juices
Brussel sprouts	Currants	Veggies Juices
Cabbage	Dates/Figs	Fresh Fruit Juice
Carrot	Grapes	Organic Milk
Cauliflower	Grapefruit	(unpasteurized)
Celery	Lime	Almond Milk
Chard	Honeydew Melon	Mineral Water
Chlorella	Nectarine	Green Tea
Collard Greens	Orange	Herbal Tea
Cucumber	Lemon	Dandelion Tea
Eggplant	Peach	Ginseng Tea
Kale	Pear	Banchi Tea
Kohlrabi	Pineapple	Kombucha
Lettuce	Papaya	Ginger Tea
Mushrooms	All Berries	Goat Milk
Mustard Greens	Tangerine	**SWEETENERS**
Dulse	Tomato	Stevia
Dandelions	Tropical Fruits	Raw honey
Edible Flowers	Watermelon	**SPICES/**
Onions	**PROTEIN**	**SEASONINGS**
Parsnips	Eggs	Cinnamon
Peas	Whey	Curry
Peppers	Cottage Cheese	Ginger
Pumpkin	Goat cheese	Mustard
Rutabaga	Chicken Breast	Chili Pepper
Romaine	Yogurt	Sea Salt
Sea Veggies		
Spinach		

ALKALIZING FOODS

		Miso Tamari All Herbs **FATS & OILS** Flaxseed Oil Olive Oil Coconut Oil Grape seed Oil **ORIENTAL VEGETABLES** Maitake Daikon Dandelion Root Shitake Kombu Reishi Nori Umeboshi Wakame

ACIDIFYING FOODS

FATS & OILS	NUTS & BUTTERS	DRUGS & CHEMICALS
Canola Oil	Cashews	Chemicals
Corn Oil	Brazil Nuts	Drugs, Medicinal
Hemp Seed Oil	Peanuts	Drugs, Psychedelic
Lard	Peanut Butter	Pesticides
Safflower Oil	Pecans	Herbicides
Sesame Oil	Tahini	**ALCOHOL**
Sunflower Oil	Walnuts	Beer
FRUITS	**ANIMAL PROTEIN**	Spirits
Cranberries	Beef	Hard Liquor
Sour Cherries	Carp	Wine
Rhubarb	Clams	**BEANS & LEGUMES**
Plums	Fish	Black Beans
Processed fruit juices	Lamb	Chickpeas
GRAINS	Lobster	Green Peas
Rice Cakes	Mussels	Kidney Beans
Wheat Cakes	Oyster	Lentils
Amaranth	**ANIMAL PROTEIN**	Lima Beans
Barley	Pork	Pinto Beans
Buckwheat	Rabbit	Red Beans
Corn	Salmon	Soybeans
Oats (rolled)	Shrimp	Soy Milk
Quinoa	Scallops	White Beans
Rice (all)	Tuna	Rice Milk
Rye	Turkey	**OTHER**
Spelt	Venison	Distilled Vinegar
Kamut	**PASTA (Flours)**	Wheat Germ
Wheat	Noodles	Potatoes
Hemp Seed Flour	Macaroni	Artificial sweeteners
DAIRY	Spaghetti	Sugar (white & brown)
Cheese, Cow	Wheat flour	Most grains
Cheese, Goat	White flour	Chocolate
Cheese, Processed	Pastries	
Cheese, Sheep		

ACIDIFYING FOODS

Milk Butter		Caffeine Coffee Tea Soft Drinks

Chapter 12
Exercise

Your skin is the largest organ of your body and perspiration is a fantastic way to aid in detoxifying the body of sickness. Exercise is imperative to rid your body of toxins and therefore you must start working out in order to be healed. The more toxins you have leaving your body, the more cancer will not have time to take hold. And, if you already have cancer, the more ways you detoxify your body, the more likely it is that cancer will leave your body. Luckily, when I found cancer in my body, I became unemployed through no fault of my own, and therefore had plenty of time to work out daily. Not that it is a good idea to be unemployed, because that increases stress levels in the body, but everything happens for a reason.

My current exercise routine consisted of ice skating, hiking, kayaking, Stairmaster, free weights, resistance machines, and anything else that I enjoyed that would burn at least 1,000 calories per day. I not only wanted to rid my body of disease, but I also had a goal to lose the last ten to fifteen pounds of fat that had taken up residence around my waistline. I am not suggesting that you take your exercise routine to the level that I had. Start out slow; if you can only manage to walk around your block once, it is a start.

When I first started at the gym, I had gotten measured by a trainer, so I could keep track of my progress. The trainer very casually said that all women want to get rid of their "baby pouch" around the middle. I told her that I did not need that "baby pouch" especially because I did not have a baby. So, my goal was to get my flat stomach back and get rid of the flabby underarms; you know what I am talking about ladies.

If the gym bores you to tears; as it does me, find an exercise plan that you enjoy doing. I had found that ice skating was fun and kept me cool, in the 110-degree heat, in the summer months. I enjoy hiking and getting out in nature because it is a great way to clear my head, pray, and just think about life. It is good to get outdoors and take in oxygen to help heal the body. It is also beneficial to exercise outdoors because I was doing the Budwig protocol, which insists on getting sunlight after consuming the mixture.

During my cancer battle, I was hiking close to fifty miles a week. Hiking is a great distraction, and it helped get me out into nature where I could clear my mind for a few hours. I would even hike in the pouring rain and still do to this day. Hiking in the rain is so cleansing and very peaceful because nobody else seems to be crazy enough to want to get wet and muddy. It is amazing how your attitude changes once you become sick with cancer. I did not mind hiking in the pouring rain because the cancer was wearing me out and I did not really care if I was hiking in mud and rain. At least then, you could not see the tears streaming down my face when the pouring rain was streaming down my face as well.

An important tip to remember while exercising is to breathe deeply to get the maximum amount of oxygen into your body. Breathe in through the nose to fill your lungs completely and then let the air slowly out through the mouth. Most people are very shallow breathers and sometimes forget to breathe when they are exercising. Make it a point to remember the breathing techniques of breathing, in through the nose and out through the mouth. This deep breathing will bring more oxygen into your cells and help to rid your body of toxins and disease quicker.

Exercise is imperative to helping the body detoxify from cancer because your body is sweating and releasing toxins. Any form of exercise is a great idea, however, exercising outdoors is the best idea because you get a chance to breathe in the fresh air and get some sunlight (hopefully). Remember to breathe deeply and get in all of the oxygen you can while you are exercising.

Exercise is key to a healthy mind and body so find an exercise routine that you enjoy doing, whether it be walking, hiking, ice skating, roller skating, the gym, swimming, or riding a bike. The point is to get out there and get sweaty as much as you can manage. Even if you can only start small with a couple of light weights at home, do what you can and do not strain yourself too much. Those with cancer also need lots of rest, so listen to your body while you are healing.

Chapter 13
Epidermal Growth Factor Receptor (EGFR)

Cancer can show itself in many forms when it is detoxing from your body. The various elimination channels are the colon, urinary tract, the mouth, nasal passages, and the skin. When I was utilizing the various cancer protocols and detoxing my body, I did experience a rash around my neck in the form of a ring. The rash had shown up a few months after I had begun the various alternative cancer protocols and eventually lasted seven months before my body was detoxed from the cancer and that is when the rash had finally dissipated. This rash was confirmed as an epidermal growth factor receptor rash (EGFR), which is indicative of cancer being within the body. You cannot possibly have the epidermal growth factor receptor rash if you do not first have cancer.

The Epidermal Growth Factor Receptor (EGFR) is "The protein found on the surface of some cells and to which epidermal growth factor binds, causing the cells to divide. It is found at abnormally high levels on the surface of many types of cancer cells, so these cells may divide excessively in the presence of epidermal growth factor." In layman's terms, it is when there is an increased layer of protein covering the cancer cell and is more prevalent in the advanced stages (stage 3 or 4) of HER1 types of cancer. You can determine your stage of cancer by the length of time you have the EGFR rash.

While I was detoxing my body from cancer, I consulted with a nutritionist, a biochemist, and various other people who had also detoxed their body from cancer. The cancer survivors had confirmed that the presence of a rash on the upper chest or neck is a sign that either breast cancer or non-small cell lung cancer is detoxing from the body. I needed to consult with these individuals because I was starting to worry as to why the rash had not went away as of yet. I was informed that the rash would not subside until my body was cleared of all cancer and the rash could last a very long time depending upon the severity and stage of cancer that I had. I had spoken to a woman who had stage 4 breast cancer who had told me that her rash had lasted just short of a year. I had also spoken to my mother, who had stage 3 breast cancer, and she said that her lymph nodes were barely swollen and didn't ache like mine. My mother also never experienced a rash, although she opted for an integrative approach, which could have impeded the natural healing process. Considering that my rash didn't dissipate for seven months and my lymph nodes were visibly swollen and constantly in pain and throbbing would put me at a pretty serious stage of cancer, at about a stage 3 or 4.

The Epidermal Growth Factor Receptor, which occurs mainly in HER1 type advanced cancer, is highly prevalent in people with non-small cell lung cancer, breast cancer, pancreatic cancer, ovarian, head and neck cancer. The EGFR is locked within the protein of the cancer cell and when released, it can appear in the form of a rash. Those cancer patients that experienced the EGFR type rash had a better survival rate than those that hadn't experienced the EGFR with a HER1 type cancer.

There is a higher survival rate in those HER1 cancer patients who experience the EGFR rash, due to the cancer being detoxed out of the body in the form of a rash. The HER1 cancer patients that don't experience the rash means that the cancer is still lurking somewhere within their cells and still needs to be released from the body. If the cancer is not released from the cancerous cell and released from the body, it will lurk in the body and eventually move to a different location.

I experienced the EGFR rash when I experienced cancer the first time. The second time, when the cancer returned, I did not experience the rash. This may be due to the fact that cancer is no longer of the inflammatory type, as it was previously, and because it is no longer in my breast or lung region. Although at certain times throughout the year, I would notice the rash coming back very faintly, as I detoxed my body, but as the detoxification progressed, the rash would dissipate. Below is a picture of me and what the epidermal growth factor receptor rash looks like, I wore turtlenecks for almost a year when I had this rash. The rash was very itchy and nothing I tried topically helped to get rid of the rash. It only disappeared after the cancer was gone.

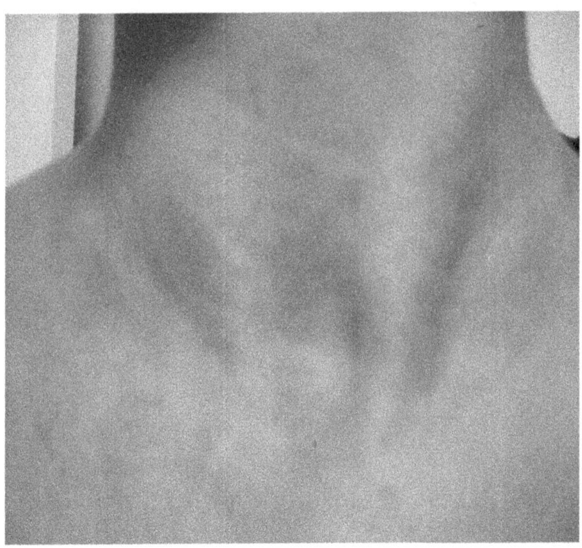

eventually move to a different location.

I experienced the [illegible] rash when I experienced cancer the first time. The second time, when the cancer returned, I did not experience the rash. This may be due to the fact that cancer is no longer of the inflammatory type, as it was previously. [illegible] cancer in my [illegible] lung region. Although a certain [illegible] year, I would [illegible] I was very faint [illegible] the [illegible] would disappear [illegible] of me [illegible] what the [illegible] turned [illegible] for almost a year when I had the [illegible] I tried [illegible] returned after the cancer [illegible]

Chapter 14
Rest, Attitude & Faith

Rest

Cancer is very draining, and you need a lot of rest for your body to fully recover. If you are tired, then you must sleep. If you are having problems sleeping, taking a melatonin supplement or valerian root tea at bedtime can help you to fall asleep faster and sleep throughout the night. Be careful with the melatonin supplements because if you take too many milligrams of melatonin, it can make you feel groggy the next day. Start with 1-3 mg of melatonin and monitor how you feel the next day before you decide to increase your dosage.

When I was in the advanced stages of cancer, I was sleeping 16 hours a day and even when I wasn't asleep, I felt as if I was in a fog and hadn't slept at all. It had taken many hours of sleep, as part of a healing regimen, to fully recover from cancer. Give yourself a break and realize that if you feel tired that your body is trying to tell you to rest, so don't push yourself or it can make you sicker. Listen to your body and make sure to get plenty of rest so your body can recover. Your immune system is trying to repair itself and is working hard to do its job at eradicating disease.

Attitude

A positive attitude is imperative to survival. If you believe you will survive and you have a will to live, then chances are great that you will survive cancer. Surround yourself with positive, uplifting people who will support you when you get depressed. Depression, angry feelings, and crying will happen because it is a sign that your body is releasing the toxins within the body. I used to cry 10 times a day, at least, for all reasons. Stay away from negative people, they will only bring you down and keep you sick.

I can't tell you how many times I was verbally attacked by horrible, negative people, who had nothing better to do with their lives than to try to attack me. What I have found is that people who are constantly negative, who will attack someone who is sick with cancer, are those people who are insecure with themselves and not worthy of your time and energy. Shake loose the negative people, even if it means letting go of your own family members, because they will impede your healing process.

All of the people whom I thought were friends, I lost when I got sick. I couldn't find many people in my life who were positive enough, so I turned to starting my own Facebook page and brought together many people who also needed support while they were sick. The great thing was that I had made more connections and met more positive people throughout the world, through social networking than any other area of my life.

It is difficult enough being sick with cancer or any disease and it is even worse when you don't have positive people surrounding you. If you have nobody in your life that is positive and supportive, go to the many websites, forums, and social networking pages, where there are thousands of people who are willing to spread the love and positivity you need to survive. Those of you who are lucky enough to have positive and uplifting people in your life, congratulations, as it makes your journey that much easier. Although, in any situation of healing, faith is an integral part that will tie the entire healing process together.

Faith

It is my personal belief that all of us have a higher power, and it is important to draw into that power to help you get well. For me, it is my faith in God. I personally turned to my faith in God to guide me through Cancer and I would pray constantly. Call in your healing and declare yourself well in the name of Jesus Christ. I also know that when life comes at you the hardest is when you are closest to victory, so keep pressing forward in faith, knowing that you will be healthy again. It is through my faith in God and reading the Bible that I realized that you can achieve Optimum Health through God's Pharmacy.

Chapter 15

What Can I Eat?

There are so many books and websites out there telling people with cancer which diet is best. All of these websites and books are confusing because most are written by people who have never had cancer and don't speak from personal experience. So, which diet works best to heal the body when you have cancer? The answer to that question is dependent upon the type of cancer, whether you have previously had cancer, which cancer diets you have undertaken previously, whether you have done chemotherapy or radiation, supplement use, and how the specific diet plan makes you feel.

I found that cancer can be caused by eating meat and dairy that contains hormones, antibiotics, and steroids. It could be because pancreatic enzymes cannot digest meat products as easily as vegetables. The digestive system becomes blocked and works less efficiently. Such foods need to be completely avoided while undertaking a cancer reversing diet.

The reason to avoid meat and dairy is because you need the pancreatic enzymes to break down the protein coating surrounding the cancer cell wall and not the protein from meat, ice cream, cheese and eggs from un-organic sources. As discussed in the chapter on enzymes, pancreatic enzymes need to be available to break down the protein barrier of the cancer cell instead of working on digesting the meat from your last meal. These enzymes are instrumental in oxygenating the cancer cells and helping them to reverse them back to normal cells.

The creation of the "Defeat Cancer Now" plan that I had utilized, combined Enzymes, The Budwig Protocol, Vitamin B17 (amygdalin), Proper Detoxification, and Juicing, it is imperative to alter your present diet and cut out all meats and dairy for a while to allow the treatments to work on the breaking down of the cancer cells and not on the food. Another reason it is important to cut out all animal products is because they create acidity in your body and will only expedite increasing cancer.

While utilizing the Budwig protocol, you must cut out all meats for the first thirty days. After that, you can re-introduce some meats, as long as they are organic. Wild fish, organic chicken, organic turkey, lamb, and organic beef would be alright to eat on occasion after being on the Budwig plan for 30 days. Although, I stayed away from meat for a year to ensure that the pancreatic enzymes, in the form of pineapple, I was ingesting were working to break down the cancer cells, and not working on breaking down my meal. I would cheat once in a while on Thanksgiving and Christmas with organic Turkey or have some wild fish and eggs, on occasion.

Many cancer patients, especially if they are in advanced stages, may have issues with their digestive system and may have what is known as intestinal permeability. This is where your digestive system is impaired by holes within the small intestines. What happens is that when you eat something, it doesn't fully digest, and whole food particles will permeate the small intestines and leak into the blood stream, which causes food allergies, auto-immune diseases, boils, rashes, and many other health conditions. In the beginning stages of intestinal permeability, it is difficult to notice, aside from a few allergic reactions to food. As your intestines become more permeable; it can lead to autoimmune diseases, extreme allergic reactions, Crohn's disease, hives, attention deficit hyperactivity disorder, inflammatory bowel disease, irritable bowel syndrome, rheumatoid arthritis, chronic fatigue, migraines, lupus, fibromyalgia, autism, ulcerative colitis, eczema, psoriasis, skin problems, schizophrenia, and celiac disease. Your stomach will also protrude, making you look pregnant when you aren't. This is due to the bad bacteria in your gut, which overtakes the good bacteria.

Intestinal permeability can be caused by antibiotic use, systemic candida, parasites, vaccines, overabundance of toxins within the body, chemotherapy, radiation, alcohol, and drug use. Due to some people having intestinal permeability, it is important to heal the gut lining if you expect to be able to absorb any nutrients from your food or supplements. You also may not be able to eat many foods due to extreme food intolerances and allergies.

I had this issue where I had to steer clear of dairy, gluten, sugars, all processed foods, hormone laden meats, and GMOs. All of these foods would cause me extreme distress with allergic reactions that would happen 10 minutes after I had eaten any of the offending foods. At first, I didn't notice the symptoms because they didn't happen too often. It became very clear later when it led to my suffering with extreme irritable bowel syndrome for an entire year. I also wasn't absorbing any nutrients that I was ingesting, and this became a problem in trying to heal my body. The best way to heal intestinal permeability is through a fasting program because it gives the intestinal lining a rest and lets it heal naturally; see the detoxification chapter for information on fasting.

During this process of trying different diet plans, I realized that not everyone can do vegan, vegetarian, or raw successfully because we all have different body chemistry. In addition to that, many of us may be in various stages of cancer that minimize the organs' ability to digest raw vegetables properly. You have to find which foods work well with your body type to reap the greatest benefits.

In August of 2011, I had a little money to be able to go to a naturopathic doctor, for blood and urine testing, where I was eventually diagnosed with low thyroid, insulin resistance, estrogen dominance, and high cortisol, just to name a few. Even though I was eating gluten free, mostly vegetables, and organic fish, I still had health issues. Many of these health issues were a direct result of detoxing from cancer too quickly, which re-released too many toxins back into my system. This created the candida to thrive, damaging my gut lining, and throwing off the balance of hormones throughout my body.

The toxic liver is one of the root causes of the cancer problems, hormonal imbalances, insulin resistance, and many other ailments. If you currently have cancer, it is a safe bet that your liver is also toxic, and you may also have a gut imbalance that needs to be corrected.

I have embraced a new way of eating which is healthier and have adopted it as a lifestyle change, which I will explain in a later chapter. I do not use the word "diet" because the word "diet" alludes to a temporary situation. You must embrace a "lifestyle change" to make it a lasting improvement in your everyday plan.

Chapter 16

The Navarro Urine Test And Additional Testing

Even though I knew that I had cancer due to the symptoms and the presence of the Epidermal Growth Factor Receptor, I still had people doubting that I ever had cancer at all because I wasn't diagnosed through the traditional method. I guess I can't blame them for being so conditioned into believing that if you don't look sick, or you haven't lost your hair from toxic chemotherapy treatments, or an allopathic medical doctor hasn't diagnosed the condition, then it isn't true. The point is, when you have advanced cancer, you definitely know it is there, there is no denying the advanced symptoms.

What most people don't realize is that there are other tests that can detect the presence of cancer within the body, even though they are not the "approved" traditional avenues of mammography, needle biopsy, PET scans, CAT scans, or MRI's. I actually had a mammogram when I was 35, when I had health insurance for a brief period of time. The mammogram couldn't be read because my breasts were too dense, although I often wonder if the mammogram isn't what propelled my breast cancer. I guess I will never know. A couple of alternative tests for cancer are less invasive and include thermography and the Navarro urine test.

Thermography is a much safer alternative to Mammograms and other archaic devices. The thermograph detects body heat, which is emitted from a malignant cell, and is very accurate at detecting cancer in any part of the body. To find someone in your area who may be offering thermography, search through the naturopathic website to find a qualified naturopath in your area at www.naturopathic.org.

John Beard, PhD and embryologist, had proven in 1902 that the trophoblast cells present in early pregnancy are nearly identical to cancer cells. Both emit the hormone called human chorionic gonadotropin, also known as HCG. HCG is the substance that protects the fetus from the mother's immune system and also protects the cancer cells. According to G. Edward Griffin, author of "World Without Cancer," "The greater the malignancy, the more these tumors begin to resemble each other, and the more clearly, they begin to take on the classic characteristics of pregnancy trophoblast."

In 1974, Dr. Virginia Livingston and her researchers also discovered the same HCG hormone existing in both pregnant women and those with cancer. According to William Fischer, "Sadly, Livingston's discovery of the growth hormone wasn't taken seriously until scientists at Rockefeller University, Princeton Laboratory, and Allegheny General Hospital in Pittsburgh isolated it in lab samples."

In the late 1950's, Dr. Manuel D. Navarro, an oncologist, had developed a test which would detect the presence of cancer within the body. The Navarro urine test is based upon the scientific theory that the trophoblast cells in pregnancy and malignant cells both display the human chorionic gonadotropin (HCG) marker. This means that cancer patients showed the same HCG markers as that of pregnant women. This test has been proven to be 95% effective in detecting cancer. The 5% of people who had inaccurate test results were of those who had "false positives" and all later had gotten cancer. Therefore, the test seems to be much more effective than 95%.

Although many people use this test to determine if their cancer treatments are working, it can also be used to detect cancer up to two years in advance. According to the Navarro Medical Clinic website, "The test detects the presence of brain cancer as early as early as 29 months before symptoms appear; 27 months for fibro sarcoma of the abdomen; 24 months for skin cancer; 12 months for cancer of the bones (metastasis from the breast extirpated 2 years earlier)." So, this would be a great method for early detection so one can change their diet and possibly avoid a future cancer diagnosis.

Dr. Efren Navarro, the son of the late Dr. Manuel D. Navarro, now runs the clinic in the Philippines and continues his father's work. When testing for the presence of HCG, to detect cancer, you must make sure that you aren't pregnant first. For women, you must abstain from sexual contact for 12 days prior to performing the test and for men; you only need to abstain for 48 hours before performing the test. If you are currently taking thyroid medication, hormone pills, vitamin D, steroid compounds, or smoke cigarettes, it is advised to stop taking these for 3 days prior to performing the urine test so it doesn't affect the results. The urine test is done at home and is very affordable and easy to do.

To perform this test, you will need:

- An unbleached coffee filter (brown)
- A glass jar
- A glass measuring cup with the cup, milliliter, and ounce measurements
- Pure Acetone (nail polish remover will NOT work)
- Rubbing Alcohol
- Measuring spoon
- Plastic sandwich bag

You may have most of these items already in your home; however, if you do not, you can purchase them for around $10.00 U.S. at your local Wal-Mart. Make sure to look in the paint department for the pure acetone, as nail polish remover will not work.

On the day of the test, take 1.7 ounces (50 ml) of first morning urine and add 7 ounces (200 ml) of acetone and 1 teaspoon (5 ml) of alcohol, put all of this into a jar and mix well. Close the jar and put it into the refrigerator for at least 6 hours, until you notice sediments have formed on the bottom of the jar. Pour off half of the urine mixture, without disturbing the sediment and re-close the jar. Shake up the sediment mixture and pour into a coffee filter to capture the sediment within the urine. Let the coffee filter air dry, indoors, until the sediment is dry. Fold up the coffee filter around the dried sediment and put into an airtight plastic bag. Then you send the sample to the Navarro lab in the Philippines, where it is tested for the presence and level of HCG.

The scale on which to measure the levels of cancer within the body are easy to read. A level of 1-49 I.U. is considered negative for the presence of HCG and 50 I.U. and above is considered a positive reading for HCG. This test will be able to tell the level of cancer within the body although it should be correlated with other test results. I highly recommend visiting the Navarro medical center website, which can be found at www.navarromedicalclinic.com to find out more information about the Navarro urine test, the cost, and address of where to send your sample.

I wish I would have known about this test in the beginning of my cancer in 2009, but I didn't. So, after having enough of the negative comments from people who doubted my having cancer to begin with, I decided to take the test to see if I still had cancer. I still felt the presence of cancer within my body due to lethargic symptoms that closely matched the symptoms I had previously, so I conducted the urine test in March of 2012, where I used my first morning urine to test. After a few weeks, I received my results via email, and this was the actual email I received from the lab:

Dear Tamara,

Your HCG Test Result on 03/31/2012 is:

Index + 4, (52.6 Int. Units)

This is within the POSITIVE range (0 I.U. - negative, 1 to 49 I.U. - doubtful [essentially negative], 50 I.U. & above - positive). A POSITIVE result indicates the presence of Human Chorionic Gonadotropin, a hormone found in the urine of pregnant women. Numerous medical reports show this to be present in the urine of cancer patients. However, the result must be correlated with the medical information (X-rays, CT scans, Ultrasounds, MRIs, etc.). A biopsy procedure confirms the diagnosis of cancer. The elevated HCG is possibly coming from remnants (microscopic or otherwise) of the breast cancer. This serves as the baseline result.

Results can go up to 10,000 int. units or more especially in testicular cancer, some uterine cancers (H mole and choriocarcinoma) and germ cell tumor. However, most other cancers have results anywhere from 50 to 80 or 90 IU. The result must be correlated with the medical history together with other pertinent medical information (X-rays, CT scans, Ultrasounds, MRIs, etc.). The test cannot determine the stage of the cancer but when it is done on a serial basis, say once a month, one can follow and monitor the progress of the disease.

Wishing you the best of health, I remain.

Sincerely Yours,

Efren F. Navarro, MD

My Test Results

According to my test results, it shows a 52.6 reading with a +4 marker. This indicates a definite positive reading for HCG (Human Chorionic Gonadotropin). Since I am definitely not pregnant, it means that I still have remnants of cancer within my body. Since my symptoms were much worse physically, with visual symptoms, in 2009 and 2010, this reading shows that the cancer is decreasing and what I have been doing thus far has been healing cancer naturally. Since I now have a positive result for the presence of cancer, I now have proof to those people who refuse to think outside of the box and realize that when cancer is in the advanced stages, there is no denying it because the symptoms are clear. Also, I knew of another cancer patient who started out in traditional methods for healing cancer when she was diagnosed with stage 4. When those traditional methods failed to work for her, she went to alternatives. She had utilized the Navarro urine test, and her number was lower than mine and she was officially diagnosed by an allopathic doctor. Sadly, the various treatments she was doing didn't work for her.

What is completely amazing is the sheer number of people who claim to be "alternative," but refuse to recognize the science and efficacy of the Navarro urine test. Also, a needle biopsy is very invasive and dangerous as it can spread cancer once that needle punctures the cancerous tumor.

Below are pictures of how to do the Navarro urine test, these are my personal samples from when I conducted the test in March of 2012.

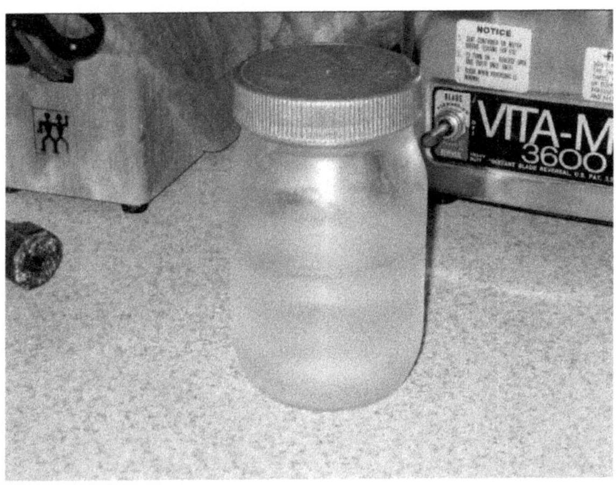

My urine Sample with sediment formed on the bottom after being in the refrigerator for six hours.

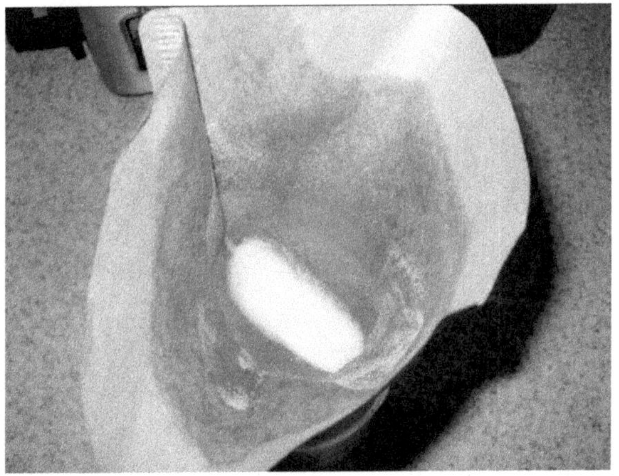

Pour the mixture into a brown coffee filter.

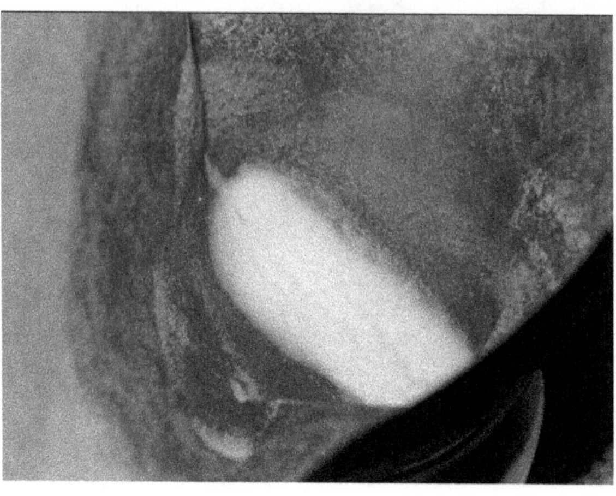

A closer picture of the sediment in the coffee filter.

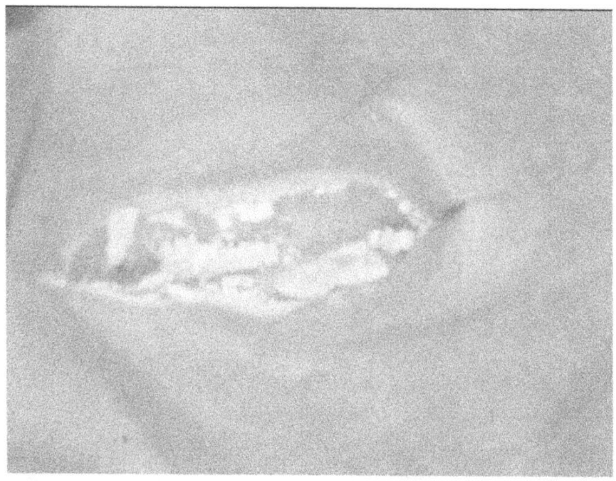

A picture of the dried sediment after it sat out on the counter for a few hours.

This is an update as of December of 2024, I kept receiving emails from various people on my social network page that the Navarro urine test is no longer available. So, I had checked with the Navarro website back then and indeed as of April 3, 2022, the Navarro clinic had requested that people not send the urine samples to Navarro clinic any longer with no explanation as to why. Now at the end of 2024 when attempting to visit the website to get further explanation, the website has disappeared.

The reason I leave this information about this testing procedure is that possibly some other clinic or doctor will begin to utilize this method in the future and also for proof of my diagnosis back in March of 2012.

As far as other testing methods are concerned. I highly suggest getting a thermography test and also getting the common blood tests for cancer. A biopsy, although commonplace amongst traditional medicine, is problematic because the needle biopsy punctures the toxic filled cancerous tumor, which can cause cancer to spread to other organs in the body. With that knowledge, it is ultimately your decision as to which testing methods you should utilize.

Chapter 17

Cancer and Disease Prevention

After finishing the detoxification program, as discussed in an earlier chapter, it is important to re-introduce necessary foods that will keep your body in perfect pH balance to increase your immune system to be able to fight off disease on its own. Vegetables are great for keeping the alkalinity up in your body and keeping pH balanced. Although, the type of vegetables and the way they are prepared are key.

It is always best to have fresh, organic produce, which is free from pesticides and that are not genetically modified (now referred to as "bioengineered"), which I discussed in an earlier chapter. To retain the flavor and vitamin content of the vegetables, do not over-cook them and never cook your food in a microwave, due to the radiation, which will irradiate your food and kill all of the beneficial vitamins, minerals, and enzymes that are necessary for good health. Irradiating your food in a microwave produces dead food and dead food in your body equal's a diseased and dead body.

Steamed or stir-fried vegetables are best for retaining flavor, vitamins, enzymes, and nutrient content. Make sure to only steam or stir fry the vegetables for a few minutes, as they are best when eaten mostly raw. Although, I am not one for all raw vegetables, so I usually steam or stir fry mine for a few minutes. If you must use oil to stir fry or cook your food, always opt for virgin coconut oil.

Virgin coconut oil contains Lauric Acid, which is beneficial for health. It is a good fat that retains flavor and beneficial enzymes at high heat and is known to lower cholesterol. Coconut oil also contains many healthy benefits, such as increased metabolism, weight loss, thyroid function, mild anti-inflammatory, antimicrobial, antifungal, antibacterial, infections, candida, gum disease, and intestinal disorders, to name a few. I will only cook my food with virgin coconut oil, because it doesn't lose its properties at high heats and it gives the food a great, mild flavor.

As I explained in the pH balance chapter, although vegetables may work to help to balance the pH level of most people, it may not work for all people due to the level of cancer or ailment and whether or not the organs are working properly. It is imperative to pay close attention to your body and test your urine pH regularly to gauge whether the vegetables are helping or harming your body.

Cancer prevention is much more effective than having to heal cancer or go through any treatments to get rid of cancer. The most important way to prevent cancer or other diseases is through your diet. Stop eating processed foods that are laden with high fructose corn syrup, genetically modified organisms (GMOs), bioengineered products, monosodium glutamate (MSG), food dyes, sugars, and various other chemicals. A basic principle that I like to use is, "if you can't read or pronounce what is on the label, it doesn't belong in your body."

Foods should contain the least amount of ingredients, so if you are buying ketchup; for example, it should only contain tomatoes, vinegar, and spices. There should be the least amount of ingredients in your food and if your food spoils quickly, that is a good indication that it is healthy for you. Our bodies are not meant to eat food with a long shelf life. It is important to eat a diet rich in organic foods with lots of fruit, vegetables, organic meats, raw milk, raw cheese, and clean, chemical free water.

Another tip to prevent cancer and other diseases is to exercise regularly to produce sweat and detoxify the body regularly in order to keep the lymph flowing and the skin clear. Your skin is a good indication of what is happening within the body, so if you suffer from blemishes, boils, cysts, eczema, psoriasis, rosacea, or other skin conditions, start by detoxing and changing your diet.

There are many people who don't see the correlation between the foods they eat and their current state of deteriorating health. Below are a few examples of parents who changed their families' diet to cut out the processed foods and GMOs and replaced it with only organic foods, the results speak for themselves.

Kayla Mason (North Bloomfield, OH)

When my 8-month-old son was diagnosed with a rare autoimmune blood disorder, our whole world was turned upside down. It has been a journey filled with many victories and losses, but tireless dedication to becoming well has granted us footing in fighting this disease. Our story is one with many details that include hospital stays, daily medication, and tremendous medical intervention to save my child's life. I want to skip that and get to what I feel is really taking my son to recovery from his ailment, diet and nutrition.

There are so many things that I didn't know when first setting out on this path of chronic illness with my son. I had never even heard of the condition he was diagnosed with, let alone the treatments or alternative treatments available for addressing it. I researched and read so much it made my heart, and my head hurt. I was drowning in information and trying to do everything on my own. Then, by grace and great fortune, I found Tamara and her online posts for Alternative Health Solutions. I wrote a message to her not knowing what reply to expect. She personally responded to me the same day and even put my concerns out for others to contribute input. The response was overwhelming for following dietary regimens like GAPS, going gluten free, and using supplements to help repair my baby's belly, which I quickly realized was our biggest culprit for much of his discomfort and even possibly the root of his disease.

Despite me telling his attending physicians that he was always bloated, seemed entirely filled with gas, screaming in pain, sometimes for days on end, all they did was assign him a nonchalant GI doctor who gave a single suggestion to stop letting him drink tea. The route to take for restoring my son's gut became very clear so I began to adjust our food choices.

Everyone associated our little family`s eating habits with being healthy, even myself, but upon closer examination, I was shocked to discover that we were not actually eating as well as previously assumed. The transformation started there; all boxed, canned, processed, GMO foods got kicked to the curb. Our shopping trips began like scavenger hunts, trying to find food without additives or gluten. This was also a little overwhelming, but transitions often are. I had the information and support I needed, and I must say that the benefits are worth the trouble.

I am a breast-feeding mom, so all dietary restrictions and allowances applied to my child, applied to me as well. Tamara really gave me the motivation I needed to go gluten free, something I felt I could never accomplish. She said plainly that I had to do it for the health of my baby. That gave me the motivation to succeed and also granted me unexpected relief from certain conditions as well.

I have always been a bit on the pudgy side, not fat, just a little soft around the edges. My tummy was always a little pooched out, which I attributed to my weight and also childbearing. I was pleasantly surprised to experience the elimination of my stomach protrusion once becoming gluten free. I know it is gluten that causes stomach bloating for me because I have cheated before and eaten some gluten only to see my familiar 3D stomach back for an appearance. If gluten did that to my belly, no wonder it would be so tough for my baby to consume it in his compromised condition.

I scrutinized ingredient lists for suspicious or modified elements, avoided all grains as much as possible, checked PLU codes for confirmation of safe growing methods, left sweeteners in the dust, forgot about processed products, and filled my shopping cart with only natural organic additive free whole foods. I make everything we eat from scratch with these quality ingredients. The changeover was challenging in many aspects, but each month, we got more comfortable and familiar with our food choices.

Recognizing real or fake food has become so much easier and even less expensive. Grocery shopping this month was a breeze! I know that I personally have more energy, high resistance to infectious diseases, and lack of digestive troubles in any form. My weight is ideal, my legs and tummy are smaller, even my feet have gotten thinner! I also have noticed improvement of the varicose veins in my legs.

My oldest son has done better by being able to focus and respond. He is part of the public-school system, which gave him a cold the very first week of school. It was like he got over one cold virus just to catch another, but his recurrent illnesses have presently been stopped entirely.

Now for the amazing and super special news about my little buddy with a blood disorder; about two weeks ago, we had our first entirely normal blood count ever! His condition had been affecting multiple components of his blood. The doctors could not fix one variable without unbalancing two or more others. Through diet and nutrition, I have done for my son what the medical community could not. I addressed all aspects of his disease, and I am confident that he will recover, not simply achieve remission.

For me, the connection to diet and chronic illness is very clear. If diet has the ability to reverse disease, it surely has the ability to prevent it. The path to health is now clearly laid out before me and I encourage everyone with whom I speak about any health affliction, to look to their diet for answers and relief. We still have a long way to go with our journey, but we are well on our way. The body is an amazing piece of machinery that is constantly working to achieve balance. Our whole being is almost entirely replaced every year by cell replication. If you commit to clean quality intake for your body, you will be rewarded with optimum wellbeing naturally. One cannot achieve Health without first moving to heal.

Bridgette Millan (CA)

After hearing about the devastating effects on children eating genetically modified foods, I was called to make drastic changes in my family's diet. Our family switched immediately to an organic diet and steered clear of genetically modified foods. Initially this was a challenge because of our comfort level with our current diet. Since then, my children have lost their belly fat and bloating in the abdomen area. They have also become more focused in school and have made noticeable changes in behavior. Their teachers have commented on how they seem more focused and well behaved. There is no doubt in my mind that the positive changes are due to the organic diet that my family has adopted. I am extremely grateful to Tamara, who opened our eyes and introduced our family to this lifestyle change.

Tyrone J. (Retired U.S. Navy, CA)

For the past three months, my family and I have been on a GMO-free diet. As a result, I have noticed a significant change in my focus, energy levels and intuition. My children have improved as well, their grades vastly improved and my children regained their childhood imagination and drive. It's a shame that we have a generation evolving through a process of genetic engineering and ROUND UP.

Chapter 18
Faith in God

The major reason that I overcame this trial of sickness, which led me to the path of wellness is not just due to changing my diet, but is also my belief, extreme faith, and trust in God. Going through the trials of life is usually when people are closest to God and turn to God for answers. During my crisis, I prayed daily, mostly hourly, and mostly through tears, that God would lead me to a treatment that would heal me of any cancer or disease lurking within my body. I had to completely give my life over to God and trust in him completely that he would heal me and lead me in the right direction.

During this trial, I figured that if it was my time to die than I was fine with that because I am a Christian and I knew that I would go to Heaven. I also believed that it didn't matter where I was; whether it is in a hospital or at home, that if God wanted to heal me of cancer than he would do so, as long as I took responsibility and the first step. So, I gave my life to God and am comfortable with my decision to forego doctors, hospitals, mutilating surgery, needles, and toxic drugs.

I made it a point to heal the way God intended, with the natural and organic plants and seeds that he had created for us to utilize for health. Everything on this earth was created by God and he created everything with healing in mind. It just takes time to find the right cure for each disease.

I now realize that most every disease and affliction is reversible using only alternative methods. I have come to this conclusion through my own trial of cancer, extensive research, experimentation, and healing.

It was also imperative for me to be close to other believers, which is why I began to attend church. I also attended a small church group and went to some healing sessions at the church. I found myself praying constantly throughout the day just to stay strong. There are so many times throughout the day that I would break into tears and feel deep despair. My faith in God has helped me through this trial and I know that God will help you as well, just ask him, he will not forsake you. Find a good church and small church support group to help you through your trial as well, it really helps to increase your faith and bring you closer to God.

Through this extremely long trial, I had faced long-term unemployment, cancer twice, deathbed once, extreme poverty, food stamps, betrayal of so-called friends, personal hate-filled verbal attacks, and hate mail. I realized that God kept pressing on my heart, telling me to write this book, to help others who are sick and also in despair. It seemed as if the longer I kept putting off finishing this book, the more horrible things kept happening to me, until I followed what God wanted me to do. I really felt a kinship with Job and his trials because my own trials were taking on a tragically similar course.

It is so easy to become lazy and complacent, especially when you are sick from cancer and trying to heal, but I had to put my best foot forward to finish this book for the Lord and hopefully to help someone in the process. Exodus 23:25 states, "Worship the Lord your God, and his blessing will be on your food and water. I will take away sickness from among you."

Healing Scriptures

It helps to remain positive through your illness and believe that you will be healed. Even though you may be very weary and feeling hopeless, it is imperative that you boost your spirit and faith by reading the bible, praying daily, or even hourly if needed, and focus upon giving your troubles to the Lord and having faith that he will heal you. Below are some healing scriptures to read daily to increase your faith and be healed in the Lord. The following scriptures are taken from the New King James Version of the bible.

Exodus 15:26 and said, "If you diligently heed the voice of the Lord your God and do what is right in His sight, give ear to His commandments and keep all His statutes, I will put none of the diseases on you which I have brought on the Egyptians. For I am the Lord who heals you."

Exodus 23:25 So you shall serve the Lord your God, and He will bless your bread and your water. And I will take sickness away from the midst of you.

Deuteronomy 7:15 "And the Lord will take away from you all sickness, and will afflict you with none of the terrible diseases of Egypt which you have known, but will lay them on all those who hate you.

2 Chronicles 30:20 And the Lord listened to Hezekiah and healed the people.

Psalms 6:2 Have mercy on me, O Lord, for I am weak; O Lord, heal me, for my bones are troubled.

Psalm 30:2 O Lord my God, I cried out to You, and You healed me.

Psalm 34:17-19 The righteous cry out, and the Lord hears, And delivers them out of all their troubles. The Lord is near to those who have a broken heart, And saves such as have a contrite spirit. Many are the afflictions of the righteous, But the Lord delivers him out of them all.

Psalm 42:11 Why are you cast down, O my soul? And why are you disquieted within me? Hope in God; For I shall yet praise Him, The help of my countenance and my God.

Psalm 50:15 Call upon Me in the day of trouble; I will deliver you, and you shall glorify Me."

Psalm 91:9-11 Because you have made the Lord, who is my refuge, Even the Most High, your dwelling place, No evil shall befall you, Nor shall any plague come near your dwelling; For He shall give His angels charge over you, To keep you in all your ways.

Psalm 103:2-4 Bless the Lord, O my soul, And forget not all His benefits: Who forgives all your iniquities, Who heals all your diseases, Who redeems your life from destruction, Who crowns you with lovingkindness and tender mercies.

Psalm 107:20 He sent His word and healed them, And delivered them from their destructions.

Psalm 147:3 He heals the brokenhearted And binds up their wounds.

Proverbs 3:7-8 Don't be impressed with your own wisdom. Instead, fear the Lord and turn your back on evil. Then you will gain renewed health and vitality.

Proverbs 4:20-22 Pay attention, my child, to what I say. Listen carefully. Don't lose sight of my words. Let them penetrate deep within your heart, for they bring life and radiant health to anyone who discovers their meaning.

Proverbs 11:17 Your own soul is nourished when you are kind, but you destroy yourself when you are cruel.

Proverbs 14:30 A relaxed attitude lengthens life; jealousy rots it away.

Proverbs 16:24 Kind words are like honey-sweet to the soul and healthy for the body.

Proverbs 17:22 A cheerful heart is good medicine, but a broken spirit saps a person's strength.

Isaiah 35:4 Say to those who are fearful-hearted, "Be strong, do not fear! Behold, your God will come with vengeance, with the recompense of God; He will come and save you."

Isaiah 40:31 But those who wait on the Lord shall renew their strength; They shall mount up with wings like eagles, They shall run and not be weary, They shall walk and not faint.

Isaiah 53:4-5 Surely He has borne our griefs And carried our sorrows; Yet we esteemed Him stricken, Smitten by God, and afflicted. But He was wounded for our transgressions, He was bruised for our iniquities; The chastisement for our peace was upon Him, And by His stripes we are healed.

Isaiah 57:19 "I create the fruit of the lips: Peace, peace to him who is far off and to him who is near," Says the Lord, "And I will heal him."

Isaiah 58:8 Then your light shall break forth like the morning, Your healing shall spring forth speedily, And your righteousness shall go before you; The glory of the Lord shall be your rear guard.

Hosea 6:1 Come, and let us return to the Lord; For He has torn, but He will heal us; He has stricken, but He will bind us up.

Malachi 4:2 But to you who fer My name The Sun of Righteousness shall arise With healing in His wings; And you shall go out And grow fat like stall-fed calves.

Matthew 4:23-24 And Jesus went about all Galilee, teaching in their synagogues, preaching the gospel of the Kingdom, and healing all kinds of sickness and all kinds of disease among the people. Then His fame went throughout all Syria; and they brought to Him all sick people who were afflicted with various diseases and torments, and those who were demon-possessed, epileptics, and paralytics; and He healed them.

Matthew 8:2-3 And behold, a leper came and worshiped Him, saying, "Lord, if You are willing, You can make me clean." Then Jesus put out His hand and touched him, saying, "I am willing; be cleansed." Immediately his leprosy was cleansed.

Matthew 8:16 When evening had come, they brought to Him many who were demon-possessed. And He cast out the spirits with a word, and healed all who were sick.

Matthew 8:17 that it might be fulfilled which was spoken by Isaiah the prophet, saying: "He himself took our infirmities And bore our sicknesses."

Matthew 9:20-22 And suddenly, a woman who had a flow of blood for twelve years came from behind and touched the hem of His garment. For she said to herself, "If only I may touch His garment, I shall be made well." But Jesus turned around and when He saw her He said, "Be of good cheer, daughter; your faith has made you well." And the woman was made well from that hour.

Matthew 9:29-30 Then he touched their eyes, saying, "According to your faith let it be to you." And their eyes were opened. And Jesus sternly warned them, saying, "See that no one knows it."

Matthew 9:35 Then Jesus went about all the cities and villages, teaching in their synagogues, preaching the gospel of the kingdom, and healing every sickness and every disease among the people.

Matthew 10:8 "Heal the sick, cleanse the lepers, raise the dead, cast out demons. Freely you have received, freely give.

Matthew 12:22 Then one was brought to Him who was demon-possessed, blind and mute; and He healed him, so that the blind and mute man both spoke and saw.

Matthew 13:15 For the hearts of this people have grown dull. Their ears are hard of hearing, And their eyes they have closed, Lest they should see with their eyes and hear with their ears, Lest they should understand with their hearts and turn, So that I should heal them.

Matthew 15:30 Then great multitudes came to Him, having with them the lame, blind, mute, maimed, and many others; and they laid them down at Jesus' feet, and He healed them.

Matthew 20:34 So Jesus had compassion and touched their eyes. And immediately their eyes received sight, and they followed Him.

Matthew 21:14 Then the blind and the lame came to Him in the temple, and He healed them.

Mark 8:25 Then He put His hands on his eyes again and made him look up. And he was restored and saw everyone clearly.

Mark 10:52 And Jesus said to him, "Go your way. Your faith has healed you." And instantly the blind man could see! Then he followed Jesus down the road.

Luke 1:37 "For with God nothing will be impossible."

Luke 7:21 And that very hour He cured many of infirmities, afflictions, and evil spirits; and to many blind He gave sight.

Luke 4:40 When the sun was setting, all those who had any that were sick with various diseases brought them to Him; and He laid His hands on every one of them and healed them.

Acts 5:16 Also a multitude gathered from the surrounding cities to Jerusalem, bringing sick people and those who were tormented by unclean spirits, and they were all healed.

Acts 9:34-35 And Peter said to him, "Aeneas, Jesus the Christ heals you. Arise and make your bed." Then he arose immediately. So all who dwelt at Lydda and Sharon saw him and turned to the Lord.

Acts 10:38 "how God anointed Jesus of Nazareth with the Holy Spirit and with power, who went about doing good and healing all who were oppressed by the devil, for God was with Him.

Acts 14:9-10 This man heard Paul speaking. Paul, observing him intently and seeing that he had faith to be healed, said with a loud voice,

"Stand up straight on your feet!" And he leaped and walked.

Romans 8:2 For the law of the Spirit of life in Christ Jesus has made me free from the law of sin and death.

Romans 8:26 Likewise the Spirit also helps in our weaknesses. For we do not know what we should pray for as we ought, but the Spirit Himself makes intercession for us with groanings which cannot be uttered.

James 5:15-16 And the prayer of faith will save the sick, and the Lord will raise him up. And if he has committed sins, he will be forgiven. Confess your trespasses to one another, and pray for one another, that you may be healed. The effective, fervent prayer of a righteous man avails much.

1 Peter 2:24 who Himself bore our sins in His own body on the tree, that we, having died to sins, might live for righteousness—by whose stripes you were healed.

3 John 2 Beloved, I pray that you may prosper in all things and be in health, just as your soul prospers.

Chapter 19

"Defeat Cancer Now" Sample Day of Therapy

The reason I wrote this book is because I know how many thousands of hours it took in research and personal experimentation to find which methods were compatible with one another and which weren't. I also know that when you have advanced cancer, the last thing you feel like doing or have time for is to research all of the alternative methods that are out there. Most people end up confused and make mistakes that can be fatal.

This is why I break down the therapies that I used to heal cancer naturally, which will make it easier for you to follow. I devised a plan that is compatible with one another and can aid in healing cancer naturally. Of course, the times are variable to your own schedule, but this will give you an idea of how to spread out the specific protocols.

If you currently have cancer, you should start with the enzymes, Budwig protocol, sunshine, juicing, coffee enemas, detoxification, organic foods, and exercise. Go slow and keep a journal to see how the plan works for you. If after a month or so, you feel that this plan may not be enough for you, you can always add in the apricot kernels to give it that added "cancer killing" boost. Although most people can do fine with the plan above, I outlined the entire plan, and you can adjust it as necessary

The reason why I say to start slow, leaving out the apricot kernels in the beginning, is to keep from having the lysing symptoms of detoxing too fast from cancer. Make sure to spread out the therapies during the day and if you begin to experience lysing symptoms, scale back and do extra coffee enemas to flush the toxins.

When starting the Budwig protocol, start slow with once a day, and work your way up to ingesting the protocol a few times per day. For the seriously ill, you may have to start with flax oil enemas to jump start your electrical system. Feel free to alter this plan to fit your needs.

4:00 am – 4:20 am:

Do Coffee enema and drink a glass of lemon water.

4:20 am – 4:45 am:

Eat a few chunks of pineapple and use "visualization" to visualize the Bromelain from the pineapple is targeting the protein layer of the cancer cell.

Eat the Budwig Protocol mixture consisting of a blended mixture of low-fat organic cottage cheese, flax oil, and unsweetened vanilla almond milk. Add freshly ground flax seed to the bottom of the dish, add a teaspoon of raw honey, layer the flaxseeds with pineapple, blueberries, strawberries, nuts, or a banana, top with the cottage cheese/flax oil mixture, and top with more nuts if desired.

I vary this by sometimes adding pineapple, banana, blueberries to the already mixed custard and add more almond milk. I will blend this to make a shake. Then get ready to go work out and sweat.

4:45 am:

While drinking or eating the Budwig Protocol, I juice greens in my high-powered blender. I drink the green juice after ingesting the Budwig Protocol.

5:00 am – 7:00 am:

Work out for one hour of cardiovascular and another hour of spot training. Lastly, sit in a dry heat sauna for at least 20 minutes for detoxification. I have been going for a five-mile hike in the mornings and then do abdominal exercises and free weights every other day. I have also varied this as to now

I am hiking about 10 miles a day to speed up the detoxification process. Hiking 10 miles takes me about 3 to 5 hours depending upon the type of hike and elevation gain.

Again, take it slow and do what you can, just make sure to get at least 15 minutes of sunlight after taking the Budwig protocol. So, if you can only manage to go outside and breathe in fresh air and take in the sunshine that is a start.

Make sure to drink plenty of lemon water to keep hydrated while working out; this will also help to flush the toxins.

7:30 am – 8:30 am:

Shower and crack open apricot kernels mixed with a bit of apple sauce to disguise the taste. Eat this along with two eggs or gluten free oatmeal. I always have the apricot kernels with organic apple sauce but sometimes vary the other part of the breakfast. As long as the meal doesn't contain meat, sugar, or salt. You can use kelp flakes or some spices to flavor your meals. You can even add cinnamon, nutmeg, and a bit of raw honey to the oatmeal. No butter or margarine allowed. Cook your food with virgin coconut oil and use the Oleolox (recipe located in Recipe chapter) for a topping. You can even add vegetables to your eggs and make an omelet.

9:00 am:

Mix together The Budwig Protocol for an after-workout snack.

11:00 am:

Do Coffee enema and drink a glass of lemon water.

12:00 noon:

Spinach salad or romaine salad for lunch with hardboiled egg, tomatoes, cucumber, with extra virgin olive oil and fresh squeezed lemon juice as a dressing. Top with freshly ground flax seeds. After the first 30 days of doing the Budwig protocol, you can add a 4 oz can of sardines packed in virgin olive oil, wild salmon, or organic chicken. But still go sparingly on the meats.

3:00 pm:

A green drink with celery, parsley, spinach, kale, romaine, cucumber, cilantro, wheatgrass, alfalfa sprouts, green bell pepper, red bell pepper, carrots, beets, two teaspoons of unfiltered apple cider vinegar, fresh lemon juice with seeds, a teaspoon of blackstrap molasses, and distilled water. Only use a few vegetables at a time.

The red pepper or carrots will add a bit of sweetness to the juice, so only use a little bit. You can also use a bit of liquid aminos to make it taste a bit better and all of this must be blended with a juicer or blender to include the pulp and the seeds which are imperative to healing. If you are making a smoothie, you will be adding water to the mix to make it more drinkable.

Please remember to vary your vegetables and don't juice the same thing every time.

5:00 pm:

Dinner consists of either a spinach salad or wild salmon and organic brown rice. You can also opt for another vegetarian meal or stir fry that is sugar free. Wild Salmon, romaine or spinach salad with a dressing of lemon juice and olive oil, steamed broccoli or another green vegetable with Oleolox.

7:00 pm:

I don't know about you, but I love dessert. I have included some Budwig dessert recipes in the recipe chapter, so you won't have to skip dessert, and you will be fighting cancer at the same time.

8:00 pm:

Drink a couple tablespoons of liquid bentonite clay to bind the toxins and it also helps you sleep more soundly. Use psyllium husk in conjunction with the Bentonite clay to increase the fiber. Melatonin supplements can also help you to sleep or drink some valerian root tea.

Make sure to drink a couple of glasses of room temperature water after taking the bentonite clay and psyllium husk to help the two expand in your body and attract the toxins to be carried out of your system.

8:45 pm:

Eat 15 Raw almonds to alkalize before bedtime and do a coffee enema.

Make sure to drink plenty of water, at least 8 glasses of room temperature water per day with fresh lemon juice added. If you are very ill, you may need to be doing at least 5 to 6 coffee enemas per day. As you start to get better, you can scale it back to 2 to 3 coffee enemas per day. The key is to flush the toxins out of your liver and your body. When you have advanced cancer, you will have a lot of toxins being released into your body as the cancer is breaking apart.

In hindsight, for someone who only has stage 1 or 2 cancers, I would opt to begin with apricot kernels, juicing, detoxing, coffee enemas, diet change. I would leave the Budwig protocol for the advanced cancer cases because it does need to be followed for five years religiously.

As stated before, this is only a general guideline for what a typical day may look like for someone trying to heal from cancer naturally. Tailor it to what you need depending upon the severity of your condition.

Chapter 20
Healthy Recipes

Budwig Protocol

Linomel

2 Tbsp ground Flax seed

1 Tbsp raw honey

Directions: In a coffee grinder, freshly grind the flaxseeds. Flaxseeds will go rancid very quickly, within 15 minutes, so make sure to eat them right away. Add the honey to the mixture. This is what will be placed on the bottom of the bowl when constructing the first layer of "The Budwig Protocol."

Flax Oil/Cottage Cheese Base Recipe

2 Tbsp Low-Fat Cottage Cheese or Quark. (Quark is more readily found in Europe, whereas the Low-fat cottage cheese is found readily in the United States.)

1 Tbsp refrigerated cold pressed flaxseed oil

1 Tbsp unsweetened almond milk, raw milk, or another unsweetened milk substitution

Directions: Add all ingredients into a container and blend using a stick type hand-held blender. Blend until smooth, where there is no oil residue left. The consistency should resemble a thick cream or custard. From this base recipe, you can add other fruits, spices, herbs but the base mixture must be incorporated first before adding anything else. This base recipe is the third layer of "The Budwig protocol."

Budwig Muesli (The Budwig Protocol)

Linomel (see above)

Budwig Base recipe (see above)

Fruit of choice (banana, apple, blueberry, raspberry, blackberry)

Chopped nuts (walnuts, hazelnuts, brazil nuts)

Directions: Add Linomel to the bottom of the bowl, layer fruit of choice on top of the Linomel, scoop the Budwig base recipe onto the fruit, and top with nuts of choice. You can also add a bit of raw honey to the top of the mix, no more than 1-2 tsp. This is great for breakfast, or anytime, and is very filling.

Oleolox (butter substitute)

8.8 ounces (250 g) virgin coconut oil

1 onion (cut in half)

10 cloves of garlic

½ cup (125 cc) Flaxseed Oil

Directions: Put flaxseed oil into a bowl and put into the freezer for 30 minutes. Put 8.8 ounces of coconut oil into a deep-frying pan over a low flame, add the onion halves and cook until both sides of the onion are slightly brown for 15 minutes. I cook the onion on one side for 7.5 minutes and turn over for the other 7.5 minutes. Add the cloves of garlic for only 3 minutes. Strain the coconut oil mixture through a fine strainer into the chilled flaxseed oil from the freezer. Discard the onions and garlic; this will give the oil the health benefits of sulphur. Keep this mixture in the refrigerator to be used as a butter replacement. Never heat the Oleolox for more than a minute. It is best to cook your food and add the Oleolox last.

Breakfast Concoctions

Scrambled Eggs

2 Tbsp Virgin Coconut Oil

2 eggs (beaten)

Directions: Heat coconut oil in pan and add beaten eggs. Get creative and add organic salsa, herbs, spices, onions, or other vegetables.

Vegetable Omelet

2 Tbsp Virgin Coconut Oil

2 eggs (beaten)

A handful of mushrooms

Chopped Green and/or Red Bell Pepper

Diced onion

½ sliced Avocado

2 Tbsp Organic Salsa or to taste

Directions: Heat coconut oil in a small omelet pan; add the onion, green/red bell pepper, and mushrooms. Sauté the vegetables until softened and add the beaten eggs. Push the mixture around the edges to the center of the pan, where the uncooked portion flows to the outer edges. Keep doing this until the entire egg mixture looks firm enough to turn over. Turn the flattened omelet over to cook the other side. You can now add avocado and organic salsa. Slide the omelet out of the pan, folding it in half to form the omelet, and onto a plate.

Soups

Vegetable Soup

3 quarts of organic vegetable broth
2 quarts of water
2 strips Kombu
1 large onion (diced)
3 cloves garlic (diced)
2 bunches of organic celery (sliced)
6-8 organic carrots (sliced)
2 organic zucchinis (bite size pieces)
1 lb. organic string beans
½ tsp Dulse flakes (or to taste)
1 tsp sea salt (or to taste)
1 Tbsp oregano
1 Tbsp Miso paste (optional)

Directions: In a 6-quart or larger pot, add vegetable broth, all chopped vegetables, and spices. Add water to fill about a couple of inches from the top of the pot. Bring to boil until all vegetables are fork tender. Ladle the soup into bowls and add some miso paste, if you wish. You can add a variation of vegetables, I usually add whatever is in my refrigerator.

Raw Spinach Avocado Soup

1 bunch Raw Spinach
1 ripe Avocado
1 tsp green curry powder (or to taste)
1 bunch Cilantro
1 tsp Sea salt or Dulse or kelp flakes (or to taste)

Directions: Put all ingredients into the high-speed blender and blend until smooth and heated through.

Butternut Squash and Sweet Potato Soup

1 Butternut squash (cut into chunks)

1 sweet potato or yam (cut into chunks)

1 15 ounce can full fat Coconut milk

3 Tablespoons of ground Cinnamon

1 Tablespoon of ground Nutmeg

½ tsp of ground Ginger

1/8 tsp ground clove

Directions: Peel and cube the butternut squash and the sweet potato. Steam both the squash and sweet potato until fork tender. Put the squash and sweet potato into the high-speed blender; add the coconut milk, and spices. Blend until smooth and heated through. If you want a thinner consistency soup, add some of the water from the steamed squash and sweet potato. If you choose not to use the steamed water, save it and drink it later to get the beneficial enzymes or add it to your vegetable smoothies. You can also substitute organic pumpkin for the sweet potato, which also makes for a wonderful soup.

Miso Soup

4-6 cups water or vegetable broth

1 sheet of Kombu or seaweed

5-6 green onions diced

2 carrots (sliced)

3 celery stalks (sliced)

2 Tablespoons barley Miso

½ tsp Dulse or kelp flakes

½ tsp sea salt

½ tsp Bragg's liquid aminos (to taste)

Directions: Bring to boil the water or vegetable broth with Kombu and diced green onions. Then put heat on simmer and add carrots, celery, Dulse flakes, and sea salt. When the carrots and celery is fork tender, add the liquid aminos, and remove pot from fire. Ladle soup into bowls and add Miso individually to the bowls. Never add Miso to boiling soup. You have to dissolve the miso paste into the soup or you will be eating chunks of miso.

Lentil Soup

This recipe is compliments of my mother, Marylee St. John.

1 cup dried brown lentils, washed and drained (Lentils do not have to be soaked before cooking)

3 Tablespoons extra virgin olive oil

1 onion, chopped

1 clove garlic, minced

2 slices bacon*, chopped (optional)

2 carrots, chopped

2 stalks of celery, chopped

1-14 oz. canned tomatoes, remove seeds

4 cups of vegetable or organic chicken stock

1 or 2 bay leaves

Salt and pepper (to taste)

Directions: Heat olive oil in large saucepan. Add bacon and sauté for a few minutes, add the onion and garlic and continue to cook and stir for about 2 more minutes. Add carrots, celery, tomatoes, lentils, vegetable or chicken stock, bay leaves, salt and pepper to taste. Bring to a boil with lid on, lower heat, and simmer for 1 to 1 1/2 hours, until lentils are tender, stirring occasionally, to prevent lentils from sticking on bottom of the pan. Remove bay leaves. If soup is too thick, thin it with a little extra stock or water. Serve hot. *Warning: Do not add bacon if you currently have cancer.

Salads

Salmon/Sardine Salad

4-6 ounces Wild Salmon or Sardines with Olive Oil
2 Tbsp Lemon juice from fresh lemons
Large handful chopped Romaine lettuce
Arugula lettuce
Spinach
1 Hard Boiled Egg (sliced)
1 Sliced Avocado
1 Ripe tomato (chopped)

Directions: Arrange lettuce in bowl, add the sliced avocado, sliced hardboiled egg, chopped tomato, add boneless sardines with olive oil on top of the salad and drizzle with fresh lemon juice. I sometimes replace the sardines with salmon leftover from the night before and then add extra virgin olive oil. Do not add the meat until 30 days of being on the Budwig plan.

Tomato/Avocado Salad

1 ripe tomato (cut into chunks)
1 ripe avocado (peeled and cut into chunks)
2 tsp of Bragg's apple cider vinegar or to taste
3 Tablespoons of Extra Virgin Olive Oil
½ tsp Basil
½ tsp Oregano
¼ tsp Dulse or kelp flakes
¼ tsp Pink Himalayan Sea Salt

Directions: peel avocado and cut into chunks. Peel tomato and cut into chunks. Put both avocado and tomato chunks into a bowl and mix the rest of the ingredients. Toss and refrigerate. Sliced cucumbers and red onions would also be a nice addition to this salad.

Main Dishes

Wild Salmon

4-6 ounces Wild Caught Salmon filets, Wild Cod, or another wild caught white fish
1 whole lemon (juiced)
3 Tbsp Coconut oil
Dill (shaken liberally over fish)
Lemon Pepper (to taste)

Directions: place coconut oil on bottom of frying pan until heated, season the fish with juice from lemon, dill, and lemon pepper and place in the pan. Cook fish for 4-5 minutes on one side and turn over for 4-5 minutes on the other side. The fish will be done when it flakes easily. You can also cook this in the broiler by putting foil on a baking sheet and grease the foil with coconut oil. Put the fish onto the foil and add more coconut oil or olive oil, lemon juice, dill, and lemon pepper. Broil for 10 minutes or until the fish flakes easily.

*Omit this dish if on the first 30 days of Budwig.

Crock Pot Stew

4 organic chicken breasts (boneless, skinless)
1 Eggplant (cut into chunks)
6 ounces of Mushrooms (or more if you like)
1 bunch Celery
1 head Broccoli
1 Onion (diced)
1 box Organic chicken or vegetable stock
1 jar Organic spaghetti sauce (no sugar)

2 Tablespoons Basil
2 Tablespoons Oregano
1 Tablespoon Cumin
1 teaspoon Sea Salt

Directions: Cut chicken into bite sized pieces. Dump everything into the crock pot and put it on high for an hour, then turn on low and simmer for 5 + hours. Make sure chicken is cooked all the way through. I usually don't measure the spices, I put a teaspoon in at a time and then alter it to taste. If you are in the first 30 days of the Budwig protocol, omit the chicken and use vegetable broth in place of chicken broth.

Vegetable Stir Fry

1 head Broccoli
1 Onion (diced)
1 Red Bell Pepper (cut into chunks)
1 Green Bell Pepper (cut into chunks)
1 bunch Celery (sliced into edible pieces)
1 Bok Choy (chopped)
1 can Water Chestnuts (sliced)
1 lb. Bean Sprouts
6 ounces Mushrooms (sliced)
8 Tablespoons Coconut Oil
Bragg's liquid aminos (to taste)
Sea salt (to taste)
Dulse or Kelp flakes (to taste)
Tamari (non-GMO)

Directions: Melt coconut oil on bottom of stir fry pan; add onions, celery, red pepper, green pepper, and bok choy. Stir fry for a few minutes until slightly tender, and then add the broccoli, mushrooms, water chestnuts, and bean sprouts. Add Bragg's liquid aminos and/or Tamari for flavor in place of soy sauce. Cover and steam vegetables until fork tender. You can also add organic chicken, wild caught fish or organic beef to this dish after 30 days of being on the Budwig protocol. Cook the meat first in the stir fry pan with the onion, take out the meat and cut into edible chunks and then add the meat and vegetables to the stir fry pan to finish cooking.

Vegetarian Chili Beans

2 16 oz cans of pinto beans
2 16 oz cans of black beans
1 16 oz can of kidney beans
1 32 oz can of diced tomatoes
1 large onion (diced)
1 green bell pepper (cut into chunks)
1 red bell pepper (cut into chunks)
1 serrano chili (diced)
1 jalapeno chili (diced)
1 yellow chili (diced)
1 teaspoon of crushed garlic
3 Tablespoons cumin
1 Tablespoon of chili powder (to taste)
1 tsp Sea salt (to taste)

Variation: You can add organic ground turkey or organic ground beef to make it non-vegetarian, but make sure that you are past the 30 days of the Budwig plan before consuming meat. You can also add a vegan meatless ground beef to this dish, and nobody will be able to tell the difference.

Directions: Chop up all vegetables and put them into crock pot. Put all ingredients into 6-quart crock pot and put on high for 1 hour, then switch to low for another 4-5 hours or longer. Make sure that all cans of beans and tomatoes do not contain added sugar. You will get some sugar from the beans, but you have to avoid the added sugars, as it will interfere with the Budwig protocol. I like my chili with a bit of a kick, but if you prefer a milder chili, omit some of the chili peppers or add a lot less. I like to either eat the beans out of a bowl or scoop them onto an Ezekiel tortilla for a healthy burrito.

Side Dishes

Mashed Potatoes

4 Russet Potatoes (scrubbed & cut into chunks)

½ cup unsweetened almond milk or unsweetened coconut milk

Directions: I sometimes leave the skins on the potatoes or if you prefer not, then peel the potatoes first before cutting into chunks. Add cut up russet potatoes to pot of water to cover the potatoes. Boil the potatoes until fork tender. Drain the water from the potatoes, keeping the potatoes in the pot. Add almond milk or coconut milk to the potatoes. Using a hand-held blender, blend the potatoes until mashed to desired consistency. Serve with a couple of teaspoons of Oleolox. Serves 2-4

Baked Potato

4 Russet potatoes (scrubbed)

Directions: Using a cookie sheet, place potatoes onto the cookie sheet and place in a 350-degree oven for 45 minutes to an hour, depending upon the size of the potato. When you squeeze the center of the potato and it "gives" a bit, you know the potato is done. Use Oleolox in place of butter. You can also add steamed veggies to the top of your potato to liven it up a bit.

Steamed Sweet Potatoes

6 Sweet potatoes or Yams (peeled and cubed)

Cinnamon

Directions: Peel and cube the sweet potatoes into bite sized pieces. Place potatoes into a steamer basket or onto a double boiler pan. Place water in the bottom pan and the steamer basket on top. Cover and boil until the potatoes are fork tender. Sprinkle cinnamon on top to taste.

String Beans

1 lb. String Beans

3 Tbsp virgin olive oil or virgin coconut oil

½ diced onion

2 sliced garlic cloves

1 tsp Dulse flakes

1 tsp sea salt

1 tsp Bragg's liquid aminos

Directions: Steam string beans until almost done. Drain the water and put string beans back into the pot. Add olive oil or coconut oil, onion, garlic, and seasoning and sauté in pan until the onions and garlic are tender and string beans are fork tender. Oleolox would also be good with this dish.

Asparagus

1 lb. Asparagus

3 Tbsp virgin olive oil or virgin coconut oil

½ diced onion

2 sliced garlic cloves

1 tsp Dulse flakes

1 tsp sea salt

1 tsp Bragg's liquid aminos

Directions: Sauté asparagus with coconut oil, onion, garlic, and seasoning and sauté in a pan until the onions and garlic are tender and asparagus are fork tender. Oleolox would also be a great addition to add the last couple minutes of cooking.

Sautéed Butternut Squash

1 butternut squash (cut into bite size pieces)
4 Tbsp virgin coconut oil
2 Tbsp ground cinnamon
1 Tbsp ground nutmeg
1 tsp ground ginger
½ tsp ground clove

Directions: Put coconut oil and butternut squash into a sauté pan and sauté until the butternut squash is almost done. Add spices and continue to sauté until squash is fork tender. This is a wonderful fall treat.

Broccoli

1 head Broccoli (cut up into bite size pieces)
Sea salt (to taste)
1 Tbsp Oleolox

Directions: Steam broccoli until fork tender. Add sea salt and Oleolox to flavor.

Brown Rice with a Kick

Organic brown rice or basmati rice
1-2 Tbsp Organic Salsa (hot, medium, or mild to taste)
1 Tbsp Oleolox

Directions: Prepare organic brown rice or basmati rice according to package directions. After cooking is complete, add Oleolox and salsa to taste.

Smoothies & Juices

Coconut Banana Pineapple Smoothie

1 can full fat coconut milk

1 ripe banana

1 cup of pineapple

1 raw egg

Directions: put all ingredients into a high-powered blender and blend until smooth. The egg adds a creamy texture. I don't add any sweetener, but you could add a bit of stevia or raw honey to taste. I find that the banana and pineapple are enough to sweeten this concoction. Serves 2 if you choose to share, but I bet you won't want to.

Green Smoothie

1 handful of raw kale

1 handful of raw spinach

2 stalks of celery

A small pinch of parsley

¼ lemon with peel and seeds

4 teaspoons unfiltered apple cider vinegar

1 Tablespoon of flax oil or freshly ground flaxseeds

Purified water to fill to top of vegetables

Optional: you may add 1 apple (with seeds), 1 pear, or some red bell pepper. Any of those would add sweetness to the green smoothie until you get used to the taste of having straight greens, no sugar.

Directions: Add all ingredients to a high-powered blender and blend until smooth. You can use these ingredients in a juicer but using a high-powered blender will keep the pulp within the juice and give you the fiber that you need to help detoxify your body.

Carrot/Beet Surprise

5 whole raw carrots
½ large beet or a full small beet
Small handful of parsley
¼ lemon with peel and seeds
4 teaspoons unfiltered apple cider vinegar
1 tablespoon of flax oil or freshly ground flaxseeds
Purified water to fill to top of vegetables

Directions: Add all ingredients to a high-powered blender and blend until smooth. If you are new to using beets in a juice, start slow with just a sliver of beet and work your way up. Beets are cleansing to the liver and too much at once can give you a "healing crisis," making you feel nauseous if you are not used to it.

Breakfast Rev-Up Juice

1 organic apple (including the seeds)
1 large grapefruit, fresh squeezed
½ cup lemon juice fresh squeezed
1 tsp organic wheatgrass powder or other green powder
Purified water to fill to top of vegetables

Directions: Add all ingredients to a high-powered blender and blend until smooth.

Vegetable Juice #1

2 large leaves of Romaine
¼ beet
2 whole carrots
2 celery stalks
4 teaspoons unfiltered apple cider vinegar

Purified water to fill to top of vegetables

Directions: Add all ingredients to a high-powered blender and blend until smooth. If you are new to using beets in a juice, start slow with just a sliver of beet and work your way up. Beets are cleansing to the liver and too much at once can give you a "healing crisis," making you feel nauseous if you are not used to it.

Vegetable Juice #2

1 handful spinach
Handful parsley
2 celery stalks
½ cucumber (peeled)
4 teaspoons unfiltered apple cider vinegar
Purified water to fill to top of vegetables

Directions: Add all ingredients to a high-powered blender and blend until smooth.

Vegetable Juice #3

5-6 carrots (scrubbed)
Purified water to fill to top of vegetables

Directions: Add all ingredients to a high-powered blender and blend until smooth.

Vegetable Juice #4

5-6 carrots (scrubbed)
¼ beet
½ cucumber (peeled)
Purified water to fill to top of vegetables

Directions: Add all ingredients to a high-powered blender and blend until smooth. If you are new to using beets in a juice, start slow with just a sliver of beet and work your way up. Beets are cleansing to the liver and too much at once can give you a "healing crisis," making you feel nauseous if you are not used to it.

Vegetable Juice #5

5-6 carrots (scrubbed)
Handful of spinach
Purified water to fill to top of vegetables

Directions: Add all ingredients to a high-powered blender and blend until smooth.

Muffins, Breads, and Crackers

Healthified Pumpkin Carrot Muffins

1 cup ground flaxseed
½ cup ground almonds or walnuts
¾ cup whey protein powder (no sugar added, chocolate or vanilla)
½ tsp baking powder
1 tsp baking soda
2 tsp ground cinnamon
1 tsp ground nutmeg
¼ tsp ground ginger
¼ tsp ground clove
½ tsp sea salt
2 tablespoon unrefined virgin coconut oil
2 eggs
2 tsp vanilla extract
2/3 cup grated carrot

2/3 cup organic pureed pumpkin

¼ cup chopped walnuts (optional)

Directions: Preheat oven to 350 degrees Fahrenheit. Line muffin tins with paper muffin cups. In a medium sized bowl, mix all dry ingredients, ground flaxseed, ground nuts, whey protein powder, baking powder, baking soda, spices, and salt. In a larger bowl, combine wet ingredients, coconut oil, eggs, vanilla, grated carrot, pureed pumpkin. Fold dry ingredients into wet ingredients until combined. Add chopped walnuts if desired and mix through. Do not over mix. Scoop mixture into the muffin cups and bake for approximately 20-25 minutes. Check with a wooden toothpick in the center of muffin until it comes out clean and dry. Store leftovers covered with plastic wrap or in a covered container in the refrigerator. Makes: 10 - 12 muffins.

Variations: Mashed banana in place of the pumpkin, pureed pumpkin in place of carrot (a double dose of pumpkin), grated apple in place of carrot, blueberry.

Healthified Blueberry Muffins

1 cup ground flaxseed

½ cup ground almonds or walnuts

¾ cup whey protein powder (no sugar added, chocolate or vanilla)

½ tsp baking powder

1 tsp baking soda

2 tsp ground cinnamon

1 tsp ground nutmeg

¼ tsp ground ginger

¼ tsp ground clove

½ tsp sea salt

2 tablespoon unrefined virgin coconut oil

2 eggs

2 tsp vanilla extract

1 cup of organic blueberries (fresh or frozen)
¼ cup chopped walnuts (optional)

Directions: Preheat oven to 350 degrees Fahrenheit. Line muffin tins with paper muffin cups. In a medium sized bowl, mix all dry ingredients, ground flaxseed, ground nuts, whey protein powder, baking powder, baking soda, spices, and salt. In a larger bowl, combine wet ingredients, coconut oil, eggs, vanilla, and blueberries. Fold dry ingredients into wet ingredients until combined. Add chopped walnuts if desired and mix through. Do not over mix. Scoop mixture into the muffin cups and bake for approximately 20-25 minutes. Check with a wooden toothpick in the center of muffin until it comes out clean and dry. Store leftovers covered with plastic wrap or in a covered container in the refrigerator. Makes: 10 - 12 muffins.

Desserts

Pumpkin Ice Cream

4 Tbsp cottage cheese
2 Tbsp flax oil
1 Tbsp unsweetened almond milk or full fat coconut milk (unsweetened)
1-2 Tbsp Raw Honey
4 Tbsp organic pumpkin puree
1 cup unsweetened almond milk or full fat coconut milk (unsweetened)
1 tsp cinnamon (or to taste)
½ tsp nutmeg (or to taste)
1 handful chopped walnuts (optional)

Directions: using a stick type blender, blend the cottage cheese, flax oil, and 1 Tbsp of almond milk or coconut milk until the mixture is a creamy consistency with no oil residue, (This is the Budwig base recipe). Then add raw honey, pumpkin puree, 1 cup almond or coconut milk and blend until incorporated. Pour ingredients into an ice cream maker and follow the directions of the machine. When the ice cream is nearly done, add chopped walnuts. If you don't have an ice cream machine, you can add the walnuts, put the mixture into a bowl and put into the freezer until it reaches an ice cream consistency. Serves: 2-4 if you want to share, but I usually eat the whole thing by myself.

Banana Walnut Ice Cream

4 Tbsp cottage cheese

2 Tbsp flax oil

1 Tbsp unsweetened almond milk or full fat coconut milk (unsweetened)

1-2 Tbsp Raw Honey

2 ripe bananas (mashed)

1 cup unsweetened almond milk or full fat coconut milk (unsweetened)

1 tsp cinnamon (to taste)

1 handful chopped walnuts (optional)

Directions: using a stick type blender, blend the cottage cheese, flax oil, and 1 Tbsp of almond milk or coconut milk until the mixture is a creamy consistency with no oil residue, (This is the Budwig base recipe). Then add raw honey, bananas, 1 cup almond or coconut milk and blend until incorporated. Pour ingredients into an ice cream maker and follow the directions of the machine. When the ice cream is nearly done, add chopped walnuts. If you don't have an ice cream machine, you can add the walnuts, put the mixture into a bowl and put into the freezer until it reaches an ice cream consistency. Serves: 2-4

Coconut Ice Cream

4 Tbsp cottage cheese
2 Tbsp flax oil
1 Tbsp full fat coconut milk (unsweetened)
1-2 Tbsp Raw Honey
1 cup full fat coconut milk (unsweetened)
1 cup unsweetened shredded coconut
1 handful chopped walnuts (optional)

Directions: using a stick type blender, blend the cottage cheese, flax oil, and 1 Tbsp of almond milk or coconut milk until the mixture is a creamy consistency with no oil residue, (This is the Budwig base recipe). Then add raw honey, 1 cup of coconut milk and blend until incorporated. Pour ingredients into an ice cream maker and follow the directions of the machine, you can add 1 cup of unsweetened shredded coconut when you put it into the machine. When the ice cream is nearly done, add chopped walnuts. If you don't have an ice cream machine, you can add the walnuts, put the mixture into a bowl and put into the freezer until it reaches an ice cream consistency. Serves: 2-4

Coconut Banana Pineapple Ice Cream

4 Tbsp cottage cheese
2 Tbsp flax oil
1 Tbsp full fat coconut milk (unsweetened)
2 Tbsp Raw Honey
1 15 oz can full fat coconut milk (unsweetened)
1 cup chopped pineapple
1 sliced banana
½ cup unsweetened shredded coconut (optional)
1 handful chopped walnuts (optional)

Directions: using a stick type blender, blend the cottage cheese, flax oil, and 1 Tbsp of almond milk or coconut milk until the mixture is a creamy consistency with no oil residue, (This is the Budwig base recipe). Then add raw honey, banana, pineapple, the rest of the coconut milk and blend until incorporated. Pour ingredients into an ice cream maker and follow the directions of the machine. When the ice cream is nearly done, add the chopped walnuts and shredded coconut (if desired). If you don't have an ice cream machine, you can add the walnuts, put the mixture into a bowl and put into the freezer until it reaches an ice cream consistency. Serves: 2-4

Blueberry Ice Cream

4 Tbsp cottage cheese
2 Tbsp flax oil
1 Tbsp unsweetened almond milk or full fat coconut milk (unsweetened)
1-2 Tbsp Raw Honey
1 cup frozen organic blueberries or another type of berry you prefer (raspberries, strawberries, blackberries, etc.)
1 cup unsweetened almond milk or full fat coconut milk (unsweetened)
1 handful chopped walnuts (optional)

Directions: using a stick type blender, blend the cottage cheese, flax oil, and 1 Tbsp of almond milk or coconut milk until the mixture is a creamy consistency with no oil residue, (This is the Budwig base recipe). Then add raw honey, blueberries, 1 cup almond or coconut milk and blend until incorporated. Pour ingredients into an ice cream maker and follow the directions of the machine. When the ice cream is nearly done, add chopped walnuts. If you don't have an ice cream machine, you can add the walnuts, put the mixture into a bowl and put into the freezer until it reaches an ice cream consistency. Serves: 2-4

Pomegranate Ice Cream

4 Tbsp cottage cheese

2 Tbsp flax oil

1 Tbsp unsweetened almond milk or full fat coconut milk (unsweetened)

1-2 Tbsp Raw Honey

4 Tbsp POM wonderful Pomegranate juice

1 cup unsweetened almond milk or full fat coconut milk (unsweetened)

1 handful chopped walnuts (optional)

Directions: using a stick type blender, blend the cottage cheese, flax oil, and 1 Tbsp of almond milk or coconut milk until the mixture is a creamy consistency with no oil residue, (This is the Budwig base recipe). Then add raw honey, pomegranate juice, 1 cup almond or coconut milk and blend until incorporated. Pour ingredients into an ice cream maker and follow the directions of the machine. When the ice cream is nearly done, add chopped walnuts. If you don't have an ice cream machine, you can add the walnuts, put the mixture into a bowl and put into the freezer until it reaches an ice cream consistency. Serves: 2-4

Chocolate Ice Cream

4 Tbsp cottage cheese

2 Tbsp flax oil

1 Tbsp unsweetened almond milk or full fat coconut milk (unsweetened)

1-2 Tbsp Raw Honey

4 Tbsp Cocoa powder

1 cup unsweetened almond milk or full fat coconut milk (unsweetened)

1 handful chopped walnuts (optional)

Directions: using a stick type blender, blend the cottage cheese, flax oil, and 1 Tbsp of almond milk or coconut milk until the mixture is a creamy consistency with no oil residue, (This is the Budwig base recipe). Then add raw honey, cocoa powder, 1 cup almond or coconut milk and blend until incorporated. Pour ingredients into an ice cream maker and follow the directions of the machine. When the ice cream is nearly done, add chopped walnuts. If you don't have an ice cream machine, you can add the walnuts, put the mixture into a bowl and put into the freezer until it reaches an ice cream consistency. Serves: 2-4

Chocolate Monkey Crunch Ice Cream

4 Tbsp cottage cheese
2 Tbsp flax oil
1 Tbsp full fat coconut milk (unsweetened)
2 Tbsp Raw Honey
2 Tbsp Unsweetened Cocoa powder
1 15 oz can full fat coconut milk (unsweetened)
1 ripe banana
1/3 cup unsweetened shredded coconut
1/3 cup finely chopped walnuts (optional)

Directions: using a stick type blender, blend the cottage cheese, flax oil, and 1 Tbsp of coconut milk until the mixture is a creamy consistency with no oil residue, (This is the Budwig base recipe). Then add raw honey, cocoa powder, 1-15 oz can of unsweetened coconut milk and blend until incorporated. Chop up the banana into pieces and add to the mix and blend until smooth. Pour ingredients into an ice cream maker and follow the directions of the machine. Add shredded coconut and chopped walnuts while the ice cream machine is running. If you don't have an ice cream machine, you can mix in the shredded coconut and chopped walnuts, put the mixture into a bowl and put into the freezer until it reaches an ice cream consistency. Serves: 2-4 if you want to share, but I am betting you won't.

Mint Chip Ice Cream

4 Tbsp cottage cheese

2 Tbsp flax oil

1 Tbsp unsweetened almond milk or full fat coconut milk (unsweetened)

1-2 Tbsp Raw Honey

1 cup unsweetened almond milk or full fat coconut milk (unsweetened)

4 Tbsp cacao nibs (sugar free)

1 Tbsp peppermint extract

1 handful chopped walnuts (optional)

Directions: using a stick type blender, blend the cottage cheese, flax oil, and 1 Tbsp of almond milk or coconut milk until the mixture is a creamy consistency with no oil residue, (This is the Budwig base recipe). Then add raw honey, peppermint extract, 1 cup almond or coconut milk and blend until incorporated. Pour ingredients into an ice cream maker and follow the directions of the machine. When the ice cream is nearly done, add cacao nibs and chopped walnuts. If you don't have an ice cream machine, you can add the cacao nibs and walnuts, put the mixture into a bowl and put into the freezer until it reaches an ice cream consistency. Serves: 2-4

Vanilla Walnut Ice Cream

4 Tbsp cottage cheese

2 Tbsp flax oil

1 Tbsp unsweetened almond milk or full fat coconut milk (unsweetened)

1-2 Tbsp Raw Honey

4 Tbsp Vanilla extract or Vanilla scraped from a vanilla bean pod.

1 cup unsweetened almond milk or full fat coconut milk (unsweetened)

1 handful chopped walnuts (optional)

Directions: using a stick type blender, blend the cottage cheese, flax oil, and 1 Tbsp of almond milk or coconut milk until the mixture is a creamy consistency with no oil residue, (This is the Budwig base recipe). Then add raw honey, Vanilla extract, 1 cup almond or coconut milk and blend until incorporated. Pour ingredients into an ice cream maker and follow the directions of the machine. When the ice cream is nearly done, add chopped walnuts. If you don't have an ice cream machine, you can add the walnuts, put the mixture into a bowl and put into the freezer until it reaches an ice cream consistency. Serves: 2-4

Vanilla Cream

6 Tbsp cottage cheese

3 Tbsp flax oil

1 Tbsp unsweetened almond milk or full fat coconut milk (unsweetened)

2 Tbsp Raw Honey

2 Tbsp Vanilla extract or the vanilla scraped from a vanilla bean pod.

1 handful chopped walnuts (optional)

Directions: using a stick type blender, blend the cottage cheese, flax oil, and 1 Tbsp of almond milk or coconut milk until the mixture is a creamy consistency with no oil residue, (This is the Budwig base recipe). Then add raw honey and vanilla and blend until incorporated. Spoon the mixture into a bowl and top with chopped walnuts for a satisfying dessert. You can also put this mixture into the freezer or an ice cream machine to make it like a creamy ice cream treat; the flax oil will not freeze, so it will stay creamy. This consistency is like pudding.

Banana Cream

6 Tbsp cottage cheese

3 Tbsp flax oil

1 Tbsp unsweetened almond milk or full fat coconut milk (unsweetened)

2 Tbsp Raw Honey

1 whole banana (sliced)

1 handful chopped walnuts (optional)

Directions: using a stick type blender, blend the cottage cheese, flax oil, and 1 Tbsp of almond milk or coconut milk until the mixture is a creamy consistency with no oil residue, (This is the Budwig base recipe). Then add raw honey and bananas and blend until incorporated. Spoon the mixture into a bowl and top with more banana slices and chopped walnuts for a satisfying dessert. You can also put this mixture into the freezer or an ice cream machine to make it like a creamy ice cream treat; the flax oil will not freeze, so it will stay creamy.

Chocolate Banana Cream

6 Tbsp cottage cheese

3 Tbsp flax oil

1 Tbsp unsweetened almond milk or full fat coconut milk (unsweetened)

2 Tbsp Raw Honey

2 Tbsp unsweetened Cocoa powder

1 whole banana (sliced)

1 handful chopped walnuts (optional)

Directions: using a stick type blender, blend the cottage cheese, flax oil, and 1 Tbsp of almond milk or coconut milk until the mixture is a creamy consistency with no oil residue, (This is the Budwig base recipe). Then add raw honey, cocoa, and bananas and blend until incorporated. Spoon the mixture into a bowl and top with more banana slices (optional) and chopped walnuts for a satisfying dessert. You can also put this mixture into the freezer or an ice cream machine to make it like a creamy ice cream treat; the flax oil will not freeze, so it will stay creamy.

Wine Cream

6 Tbsp cottage cheese

3 Tbsp flax oil

1 Tbsp unsweetened almond milk or full fat coconut milk (unsweetened)

2 Tbsp Raw Honey

2 Tbsp organic wine

1 handful chopped walnuts (optional)

Directions: using a stick type blender, blend the cottage cheese, flax oil, and 1 Tbsp of almond milk or coconut milk until the mixture is a creamy consistency with no oil residue, (This is the Budwig base recipe). Then add raw honey and wine and blend until incorporated. Spoon the mixture into a bowl and top with chopped walnuts for a satisfying dessert. You can also put this mixture into the freezer or an ice cream machine to make it like a creamy ice cream treat; the flax oil will not freeze, so it will stay creamy. You can also substitute organic champagne for the wine, as both are allowed in moderation on the Budwig protocol.

Chapter 21
Testimonials

The following testimonials are from real people who had been diagnosed with cancer. Some had used surgery, chemotherapy, and radiation before finding out about alternatives. All attribute their success in healing to utilizing alternative methods of treatment. Some people have chosen to remain anonymous. Within these testimonials there are various methods of healing because not all treatments may work for each individual.

Maurene Mongan (San Diego, CA)

"Tamara St. John was (and still is) my lifesaver. I don't think I'd be where I am today (CANCER FREE) without her help and guidance. After being diagnosed with breast cancer in March 2010 and I immediately became a vegan. I knew I had to make some drastic changes in my lifestyle because I knew I wasn't going to go the conventional route of chemo, surgery and radiation. I walked out of the hospital and never turned back.

I spent the next year and a half trying everything. I would jump from one thing to another and spend so much money on supplements that I really didn't need. I drank so many green drinks that I actually turned green. Blond hair and green skin (not a pretty site). I did shrink my cancer but couldn't continue on the massive green drink path much longer.

I sat at the computer and researched pretty much day and night. One day in my web searching something came up with Tamara's name and link to her website. Of course, I clicked on it and as soon as I read her Bio and how she healed herself I knew I needed to call her for a consultation. And the rest is history. What I had been looking for was someone to tell me what to do and guide me through the process. I'm someone who needs a plan of action and that's exactly what Tamara gave me. I spent hours (and still do) on her Facebook page where she shares amazing information. And the most important thing that I love about Tamara - she really truly cares. I know 100% that I am cancer free because of the guidance from Tamara St. John!"

Keri H (Long Beach, CA)

In 2005 at the age of 30, I was diagnosed with stage 2 breast cancer. Because of how young I was for breast cancer, according to the doctors, they were ready to act fast. I perceived that I was healthy being a practicing vegetarian for 10 years already during that time so how could I have cancer? I was shocked and stunned and the doctors gave me no time to think.

Three weeks after my diagnoses the doctors had performed a double mastectomy with several lymph nodes removed where 15 tumors were found, and cancer had already spread to my lymph nodes. Right after surgery is when I learned that I was highly allergic to all pain medication, Yikes! That was just the beginning of the downward spiral of what modern medicine has done to my body.

One month after the removal of my breasts and several lymph nodes, I was put on three types of the most aggressive chemotherapy for 6 months, which felt like it lasted for an eternity. During that time, I had really bad reactions to all of the medication learning how sensitive my system is to all prescribed and conventional drugs. It was sheer hell.

During that down time, I had learned that my cancer was 99% estrogen positive which turns out all the tofu and soy products I was overindulging in had a large part in creating the cancer. There really is something about the over processed foods and GMO products that's been produced in our country. The cancer I developed was a result of that.

About after a year and 9 months of surgeries, chemo, and other prescribed drugs, the doctors released me back into the normal world to live a "normal life" with no instructions on how to overcome what I just went through or even how to properly take care of myself to prevent cancer from happening again.

I tried to get back to a somewhat normal life and swept the traumatic incident under the rug as if it never happened, but life did not feel normal. I didn't realize that I had developed Post Traumatic Stress which included major anxiety and depression. I did not feel healthy, I struggled for energy, hid in my house, and isolated myself because I could not relate to anyone else it seemed.

Then 5 years after going through cancer the first time, I felt a hard lump in my armpit. I knew what it was and went into denial for 6 months. During those 6 months I drank heavily trying to self-medicate myself because I did not want to face cancer, doctors, or treatments again. Finally, I got out of denial and went to the doctors. I developed cancer in my lymph nodes again. The plan was to have more lymph nodes removed, more aggressive chemo, and added radiation. I was in complete and utter fear.

I wanted to go the natural approach which I had shared with my family, and they flipped. Family members made threats to force me into the hospital for treatment upon learning that I was going to refuse chemo/radiation. I understand these reactions were all done out of fear, but it was a huge unnecessary stressful battle. I opted for the surgery to make a compromise with my family. This was a very, very poor decision since operating only makes cancer spread more. I had the surgery and ate clean for 9 months, but unfortunately had a lot of anger. I couldn't heal with all that anger.

After 9 months of eating clean and being angry, I went back into denial and resumed eating processed foods, drinking alcohol, etc. just as if nothing happened. I was very unhappy and scared. Then gratefully through a friend I had learned of Tamara and her story. We became friends on Facebook during the time of Tamara's healing from cancer and developing her book. Tamara was a light in the dark place I had been in for so long. She really got the wheels turning for me on the subject of properly healing from cancer naturally.

I was also grateful and blessed to meet a friend who was a student therapist practicing how to treat people with Post Traumatic Stress disorder using EMDR treatments which work amazing well and I highly recommend it to everyone. EMDR treatments helped me to overcome my anger of having cancer and other things which have helped me to get on board with healing.

Right when Tamara had published her book I was finding out that I still had cancer which is was now stage 4 cancer that had spread from lymph to bone at the age of 38. I bought Tamara's book, Defeat Cancer Now, and studied it and did research. I am very happy to share with you that I am now into day 101 of healing naturally from stage 4 cancer and I am committed with very little fear. The only thing I fear is the doctors and the medical system.

I followed Tamara's instructions on how to properly cleanse the organs in the right order. IT WORKS!!! This is the best I have felt in years. Cleansing has been so interesting, and I see and feel how well it works and highly recommend it to others. One of my favorite things that I practice each day that I have really seen much improvement with is coffee enemas. I cried the first time I did it, but it is really easy once you get over the fear of it. I had such a dirty system and organs and can't believe how much toxins can get crammed packed in our body. It is mind blowing. I LOVE eliminating the toxins now that I know how to do it thanks to, Defeat Cancer Now.

Along with cleansing the organs, eating clean, getting proper rest and exercise. I am also using the apricot kernels, Essiac Tea, and just recently started the Budwig Protocol. I feel great! I am dedicated to eating clean for the rest of my life and am confident that I will heal from cancer completely. My body feels lighter as well as clearer thinking and a more positive outlook on life.

I couldn't have done this without the encouragement of Tamara and the guidance of her book. I am very grateful to Tamara. I would just like to add to never compromise your health for anyone and please steer away from processed soy, foods, and GMO products. I wish you great health and healing because it is an awesome adventure!

Jane Doe (Seal Beach, CA)

This is a great testimony of an 88-year-old woman from Seal Beach, CA. She preferred to keep her name anonymous. She was diagnosed with Stage III Breast Cancer in late 2011. This 88-year-old woman had attended my Alternative Health Solutions Seminar with her son, where I spoke of the alternative treatments that I used to heal cancer naturally, specifically The Budwig Protocol.

After hearing me speak, she had decided to begin utilizing the Budwig Protocol for her cancer. She had 3 tumors in her breast, one the size of an egg. She had the large tumor removed and began the Budwig Protocol. Initially the Oncologist had wanted to do radiation after her surgery. However, when she returned to the oncologist two weeks later for the pre-op MRI for the other tumors, the oncologist couldn't find the tumors. They had disappeared!

Not being able to understand what had happened, the doctors sent her to a different MRI center, to confirm the results, and again no tumors were found. All radiation treatments were cancelled, and she has only had follow-up MRIs since that time along with the Hormone Therapy to reduce her estrogen level, which she finished in March of 2012. The Oncologist and her General Practitioner both were astounded, and then her son explained to the doctors about the Budwig Protocol and both doctors were researching it as they left the Oncologist's office.

In April of 2012, she had a follow up MRI, and everything on both breasts showed negative for any cancer of any kind. More proof that alternative treatments are extremely effective, and you can achieve optimum health through God's Pharmacy.

Marylee St. John (Rowland Heights, CA)

My nightmare began when I found a lump in my breast, while sleeping on my stomach. When I went to the doctor, he could not find the lump, and he said that mammograms are dangerous and suggested that I do not get one. When I got home, I tried to find the lump while lying on my back, I could not find it, but I could find it while lying on my stomach, which is why the doctor could not find the lump. So, I quit sleeping on my stomach and forgot all about it, in other words, I was in denial. This lasted for a year in a half, and then the lump started hurting, so I decided to try another doctor. He had me take a mammogram, and then a biopsy; it showed I had cancer, estrogen related.

I had surgery and they removed 18 lymph nodes, 17 out of the 18 were positive that the cancer had spread, and it was stage 3. I went to seven different oncologists for advice, since I had a bad diagnosis. Six of the seven said that I had a 25% chance of making it 5 years, and one told me that I had NO chance of making it 5 years. So, I picked the oncologist who had a more positive attitude about my case.

The oncologist advised 2 years of chemo and then radiation treatments, he then added on Tamoxifen for 8 years, because the cancer had spread to so many lymph nodes. I quit the Tamoxifen before the 8 years was up, and did not tell my oncologist, I do not suggest that you do the same.

After a few chemo treatments I found out about alternative ways to treat cancer, so I did the Concord grape juice diet for 6 weeks. It turned my teeth black, and the dentist had a hard time getting them white again. That probably happened because I ate a lot of lemons all my life, which removed a lot of the enamel on my teeth. After the grape juice diet, my brother gave me a book titled “One Answer to Cancer” by Dr. William Donald Kelley. After using his method of curing cancer, I saw a program on T.V., with Dr. Ann Wigmore, from Boston, Massachusetts, talking about natural methods for beating cancer, and so I attended all of her lectures.

I learned a lot from Dr. Wigmore, she taught us how to juice wheatgrass, juice carrots and parsley, sprouting, coffee enemas, the importance of enzymes, and much more. After that cancer diet, I went on the Gerson diet, juicing, basically almost the same as Dr. Ann Wigmore's program. I did about 5 or 6 different cancer diets, one right after the other; I guess I was pretty scared.

My husband said that I was doing so many different diets, that I wouldn't know which one worked; I said I don't care, just so one works. After all I had to finish raising my two small children, and that was my job, not someone else who would not love them as I did. Someone gave me a tape of Jesus and His healing light going through your body and healing you. So twice a day I would lie down on my bed while it was quiet, listening to the tape and visualized Jesus going through my body with His healing light touching every part of me.

When I told the doctor, after just a few chemo treatments, that I was going to detoxify my body and go on with an alternative method, he told me to wait until after all my chemotherapy treatments were completed. I did not listen to him, I felt that this was helping me more, so I prayed "Lord if I am really healed, then when I go for my next chemo treatment, let the doctor cut me down to one year instead of the two years of chemo", and guess what, he did.

After my chemo treatment was over I was to take radiation treatments, so I was sent to the radiologist for a consultation, the radiologist was all bent over and deformed, he said that he had gotten that way from working around too much radiation, so I got scared, but I did let them set up an appointment for me to have the treatments. The next time I saw my oncologist, I was to have my first radiation treatment in the next room, once more I prayed (because I was afraid of radiation) "Lord, if I am really healed, then when I go in to see my doctor, let him forget about giving me the radiation treatments". And guess what, after my office visit my doctor never mentioned about the radiation, and I went home without the treatment. I saw him for over

16 years, and he never even once mentioned it and I never had even one treatment, he really did forget. Thank you, Jesus.

Twelve years after I had breast cancer, I got another cancer, parotid gland cancer; it had also spread to my lymph node. That's a long story, so if I decide to write a book, I will tell my story. One more thing, my husband was right, I did so many cancer diets, that I did not know which one worked for me. So, I started with the grape juice diet again, then did Dr. Donald Kelley, and combined it with Dr. Ann Wigmore's diet. I did not take any chemo or radiation at all with parotid gland cancer.

November 2012, I will be cancer free of breast cancer for 29 years, and the parotid gland cancer for 17 years. I get very fearful when November comes around, since both cancers were found in November. After all these years my oncologist told me that I proved all those doctors wrong. Praise be to the Lord.

**This is an update as of December of 2024 written by Tamara St. John, daughter of Marylee St. John. Sometime back in 2016, my mother had found out that cancer came back for a third time to her bones. My mother started on the protocols in this book and was faithfully doing everything and the doctors were amazed that she was still living. She had refused all traditional medical treatments of chemotherapy and/or radiation. She was doing well as her and I took a long trip to Europe in September of 2017, as it was a dream of hers and mine to visit Italy. When she returned from the trip, she still continued to eat right for a while but was getting tired of doing all of the protocols (i.e., Budwig, juicing, apricot kernels). My mother never got into the detoxing phase other than detoxing naturally via juicing. Sometime in 2018 was when she decided that she didn't want to fight cancer any longer, she was 79 and pretty tired of always having to eat right, juicing, and everything else. Those of you who have been through cancer may know what I am talking about? I remember myself thinking how exhausting everything was, you are already exhausted from cancer and then having to constantly juice or make meals and juices gets to be a bit much, especially when you live alone and have no help. The doctors were amazed she had lived so long, as their original diagnosis was that she wouldn't live longer than a year. By the beginning of December of 2019, my mother was 81 and went to be with the Lord on December 8, 2019. I don't blame her for stopping all the juicing. In her last year, she just wanted to eat whatever she liked and of course that included foods that were not good for anyone with or without cancer. My mother had lived a long, good life and fought cancer head on many times.

When it comes down to it, we all make a choice as to how we want to live and how we want to die. She chose to stop fighting and meet Jesus and nobody can blame her for that. See you in heaven mother. With Love, your daughter Tamara.

Naomi Havens (Richmond Hill, GA)

The day after Christmas 1999, I began running a fever which lasted about a month and had a feeling like a lump was in my throat at shoulder level. The only thing I could think of might be causing this was all of the sugar I had consumed on Christmas day, which really wasn't any more than normal. My husband was recently unemployed, and I struggled with going to just any doctor, so I tried doctoring it myself using Pau D'arco, an aromatherapy solution made with spearmint, lavender, tea tree, and myrrh. I was also using aspirin, which kept the fever down and allowed me to get through my day normally.

After the fever went away, I was left with a lump feeling in my throat. For several months, I experimented with different foods, specifically chocolate and sugar, to see how the lump was affected. As long as I avoided chocolate and sugar, the lump did not bother me much. I splurged periodically.

In June of 2000, I noticed a lump located about 5 fingers above my right nipple. I also noticed I was beginning to experience night sweats, but thought I was beginning menopause. At this time, my family and I had just moved to a new area, so I began looking for a doctor to check the lump in my throat, as well as the lump above my breast. One doctor took a throat culture to see if the lump in my throat was strep throat; I knew it was not. He ordered a mammogram, but I was not pleased with him, so I began searching for another doctor. By the time I found a doctor I might like, our family was moving again, back to where we had been 9 months prior.

I immediately began pursuing an appointment with a doctor I had heard many good things about. It took several months, but I finally got in. In January 2002, I was diagnosed with breast cancer and had a lumpectomy right away. I was told that microscopically, the tumor was poorly differentiated or grade III and measured 2.1 cm making it a T2 tumor. The tumor did not express estrogen or progesterone receptors. Two of my three layers of lymph nodes were removed and declared clear of cancer. A nerve was cut in order to reach one layer of lymph node, causing me to be numb in my armpit and the underside of my arm from my shoulder to my elbow.

Initially, due to my lack of knowledge about any alternatives (which my gut feeling told me there must be something); I planned on going the chemo and radiation route but was not comfortable with the idea. I know many people who have successfully done chemo and radiation seemingly without long-term complications. I also know people, including an aunt of mine, and my grandfather, who did not have complication-free experiences, or died during treatment.

A friend reminded me of the book "Hope When It Hurts" written by Larry Burkett, a cancer survivor. My husband and I began reading it, sometimes while waiting to see the doctor (one time while waiting for the doctor to return to the room between five phone calls). This book opened our eyes to what chemo and radiation really are. It also introduced us to an alternative therapy, AM-2, which has been used for many years for many types of cancer, including breast.

We also researched other alternatives but felt AM-2 was the best route for me. Part of that decision was due to watching my grandfather, who had been over radiated, causing his body to not be able to manufacture blood cells properly and lead to him needing blood transfusions every 4 weeks. Just before I began the AM-2 treatment, my grandfather began receiving immune boosting shots, which gave him renewed energy. AM-2 is an immune boosting therapy, whose intent is to build the immune system and help it to be strong enough to fight off cancer, as well as other attackers. The treatment involved regular IV treatments (one per day for 20 days) as well as following a strict diet, which puts a big emphasis on fruits and vegetables as the main food, along with drinking lots of water. This made sense to us.

I wrote letters to both the surgeon and the oncologist, expressing my respect for them and their positions, and then informing them that I would not be going their route. They sent certified letters telling me that if I did not go their route, I'd be dead within 5 years. They also sent letters to my general practitioner trying to get her to force me to go their route. I thank God that she stood up for me telling them that I was an adult, and that I could make the decision myself.

I do want to mention what I believe was an angel sent from God in the form of a nurse. This nurse was responsible for taking my vital signs in preparation for my initial interview with a radiologist. When I shared my concerns and preference, she replied "No one can make you do what you do not want to do." This statement gave me the confidence to pursue the alternative route I felt God was asking me to take.

In late February 2002, with the assistance of a local naturopathic doctor, and believing I had a 50/50 chance with chemo and radiation and a 50/50 chance with an alternative treatment, I began the first round of AM-2 IV treatments. I saw immediate help – I was having problems raising my arm higher than my shoulder after the surgery. After the first 2 or 3 AM-2 IV's, I could raise my arm straight up with no problems or pain.

Six months later, approximately September 2002, I went through a second round of AM-2 IV treatments, as recommended. There was confusion about some of the diet protocol, as well as how long I should continue with AM-2. The naturopathic doctor was experimenting on me, as she had not heard of the therapy until I introduced it to her, so had no real direction to point me in. Also, the state of Georgia does not recognize the naturopathic license, so this doctor had to practice under a state licensed MD, in this case, a pediatrician who integrates conventional medicine with Chinese medicine. He was unfamiliar with AM-2 as well.

In addition to the AM-2 treatment, watching my diet, drinking lots of distilled water (approx. ½ gal. per day); I was regularly juicing carrots and taking a variety of supplements including Barley Green, Juice Plus Orchard & Garden Blends, and others. By the way, the cost for the AM-2 was not covered by insurance, so it was all out-of-pocket, and was not cheap.

In July 2003, I experienced a great deal of stress at work and had slipped back into eating poorly. During this time, I felt the stress settling in my surgery area causing a feeling of swelling. I had a blood test done and, depending on the results, planned to do another round of AM-2. The blood test said my cancer levels were within normal range (as they had shown every 3 months since surgery), so for financial reasons, I canceled the AM-2 treatment. A couple of weeks later I was still experiencing the feeling of swelling, even though the stress at work had died down. I then began feeling like something was blocking a nerve or something in my arm causing increased irritation. Soon after, I found a lump approximately 3 fingers from my nipple.

In October 2003, I had a mammogram and sonogram done, which showed an abnormality (I had been trying to tell the doctors something was wrong). In November 2003, a biopsy was done, which showed the lump was cancerous. The surgeon wanted to do a mastectomy, chemo and radiation, but I was not interested in that route.

I had begun doing a lot of reading about cancer and alternatives. A lot of the information I read seemed to enforce the idea of treating the immune system, as well as having more of a vegetarian diet. Being a meat and potatoes lover, as well as never before having to watch what I ate, I really struggled with eating a proper diet.

The naturopathic doctor was no longer an option, as the pediatrician she was under became concerned that he would lose his practice due to the amount of cancer patients who were beginning to come to their clinic. So, we were dropped like a lead balloon with no direction as to where to go next.

Other therapies I tried were: The Rife Machine, Dendritic Therapy, The Blood Type Diet - which was very limiting and difficult for me to follow, Hallelujah Diet - which was so different from what I was accustomed to that I followed some of the guidelines but continued to eat similar to how I was raised. More recently I also did the Dendritic Cell Therapy. I am now embracing the Hallelujah Diet as the only way for me.

In 2005, I learned about a therapy out of Germany, called Carnivora, which is made from compounds found in the Venus Fly Trap. It comes in two forms – one for injecting directly into the tumor, the other for dropping onto your tongue. I began using the injectable form but ran out quickly both of it and of money for it. My husband's brother's dentist told him that he had bought the Carnivora drops and had some left that he wanted to get rid of. We were able to purchase it at a discounted rate. I began dropping it on my tongue, but one morning got the bright idea, "This is liquid Carnivora just like the injectable form I was using, so why not inject some of this!" Within 15 minutes I found out why not – the drops are much more concentrated. I unintentionally overdosed, which caused me to detox way too fast. My kidneys felt like they were going to explode, and the toxins landed on my lower right back.

I had to quit my job. For the next six months I lived in excruciating lower back pain and went from doctor to doctor trying to figure out exactly what was happening in my back. My gut told me I had toxin build up, but doctors were concerned with metastasis. I had test after test and ingested more radioactive compounds than I ever wanted to, only to have the test results be lost. I wrote those doctors off!!

One chiropractor tried to force me into an adjustment; I no longer go to him or recommend him. Another chiropractor, the one I've been seeing since then, suggested I do a coffee enema. The coffee enema sounded way too gross, and I thought "what does he know about cancer?", so I did not try the enemas.

While doing research in 2005, my husband began learning about the toxins in our mouths due to dental work. My mouth was full of dental work, and most of it contained mercury. The research showed promise in being able to help clear up the issue in my lower back, as well as the cancerous tumor I was carrying, so we flew to California to interview some doctors in Tijuana about removing all my teeth. A couple of months later I had all my teeth removed. They also scraped the jawbone to try to remove any mercury shadow that might be in it. I had a little relief from my lower back pain, but not much.

In September 2005, I was in so much lower back pain that getting out of bed was a 15-minute ordeal, and no one could help me because if they tried, they may unintentionally pull me in the wrong direction causing excruciating pain which would cause me to have to lie back down and wait for it to subside.

After more research, the decision was made to go to the Cancer Treatment Center of America in Tulsa, OK. At CTCA I went through more tests and was given an unending prescription for Oxycodone for my lower back pain, which only made the pain manageable & had the potential for me to become addicted. Doctors there could not figure out what the issue was in my back and were more focused on the tumor in my breast. At one point they informed me that they would not pursue my lower back issue any further until I allowed them to do a mastectomy. I really wanted to find a way to naturally take care of the tumor, but was desperate for back relief, so agreed to the mastectomy. During my recovery after surgery, I began doing Epsom salt detox, where I would drink an Epsom salt mixture. I began experiencing small amounts of temporary lower back pain relief, which confirmed in my mind what my gut had told me earlier in the year – I had detoxed too fast and was dealing with infection from that.

While checking out of CTCA I was instructed to come back in two weeks to begin radiation on my lower back. WHAT!! They couldn't determine what was going on with my lower back, yet they wanted to start radiation on it? I never went back.

While at CTCA my husband continued to research. Soon after returning home, he found a former radiologist who was now treating patients with the AM-2 that we had experienced success with. She had successfully treated herself with AM-2, which caused her to quit the radiology job she had held for 17 years. So, I began making twice a year eleven-hour drives to stay in a hotel, out-of-pocket, to be treated by this doctor over the next four years. She was my life saver!! She was my support system, of which I was desperate for as my own church & local community had failed to do. She also instructed me to begin coffee enemas every day after each IV treatment to help rid my body of the toxins that the AM-2 was releasing. Within three coffee enemas my lower back issue was cleared up, and I quit the Oxycodone cold turkey!! Just think, if I had done the coffee enema back when my chiropractor suggested it, I would still have all my natural teeth and would still have my right breast. This wonderful doctor retired and no one experienced and knowledgeable like her was left to take her place. So, I've had to stand on my own two feet and be my own doctor.

It has been a process of getting my mind and taste buds to cooperate with this new lifestyle and way of eating, but I can now say that I am finally comfortable in my own skin and with the journey God has asked me to take.

In high school the prophet Daniel became my favorite Bible character because of his determination, as a teenager, to not defile himself. At that time, I had no idea that my journey would be so close to his. I've struggled with the lack of support, and even thought about suicide. But in 2010 God introduced me to the song "More Beautiful You" by Jonny Diaz. In that song, God wrapped his arms around me and gave me the will & confidence to live in spite of what is going on around me. God also used that song to ask me to start a non-profit with the purpose of coming alongside others pursuing alternative therapies, so they don't have to do it alone like I did.

In 2009, I was following a vegetarian diet, eating lots of cheese and fish, which I loved both. In December 2009, I decided to take the vegan plunge. Within two weeks of taking the plunge, I began receiving comments from acquaintances, as well as total strangers, about how healthy I looked. I have been vegan ever since and am perfectly comfortable with it. To this day I still receive comments about how healthy I look. My blood work has improved, and I can confidently say that I am totally cancer free.

My current challenge is to eat more raw foods. Homemade green smoothies are a staple in my diet, but I'd like to get into the habit of making many of the raw recipes that are in the books I collect and on the websites I visit. Thanks for letting me share!

Co-founder & CEO at Victory Haven, an Alternative Cancer Support & Assistance Group.

www.VictoryHaven.org

Marlene Farley (Lake Charles, Louisiana)

My story began 5 years before my diagnosis when my grandmother was faced with the decision to do chemo or not. It was her third time to have cancer but her first time to do chemo. The Dr's promised her a little more time if she did the chemo and I was stuck in CA in a custody battle. She told me she was going to do it because she wanted to see my kids one more time. That was our last conversation. She did one IV chemo and got horribly sick and was gone in just 7 days leaving me to fly home on my birthday for the funeral without my 4 younger children. I was forced to leave them with their mentally ill father. It was heartbreaking and tragic. From that moment, I said to many people that if I ever had to make that choice, chemo would be a hard no for me.

Fast forward to Feb 15, 2005, when I was diagnosed with aggressive stage 3 breast cancer. The doctors came into the room and said, "your lumps are not benign." And not only that but the doctor followed with the idea that I would need to go down the hall immediately to begin chemo. I said, to their shock and disbelief, "I am not doing chemo today or any other day." That particular doctor got so flustered that I could see her blood pressure go up. She told me that anyone who survives without chemo is "damn lucky". She then left the room and came back with two more doctors who tried their best to persuade me to go down the hall to begin their toxic torture. One of them looked at me and said, "You don't even love your children!" I had 7 children at the time who I absolutely adored and were my whole reason for waking up every day. I didn't respond much to them other than to continue saying no. They then brought me down the hall to belittle me further and brought in yet more doctors and the head of oncology. I was done. I stood there with my arms crossed and rolled my eyes as the doctor began to spew more of the same garbage. He then told me to get that smirk off my face and that I was wasting his time. I said, "No sir, you are wasting my time. Can I leave now?"

Driving home from that appointment, I spent my time on the phone letting everyone know the diagnosis and assuring them that I would be fine. Knowing that chemo was never going to happen, I still had to make the decision about radiation, drugs, and surgery. After many weeks of praying, I decided to forgo radiation and drugs and go ahead with a modified radical mastectomy on the left side. Having 8 out of 14 positive lymph nodes pushed me forward into the surgical decision. I made an appointment with a very wonderful doctor in Baton Rouge, Louisiana. My doctor fully supported my decision to use alternative treatments. He did, however, strongly encourage me to have radiation which I later refused.

The mastectomy went well, and I began my own treatments. I purchased an infrared sauna because it will detox heavy metals and other toxins from the body. In addition to the almost daily use of the sauna, I ate only raw vegetables for 5 months, did organic coffee enemas, and took a large amount of supplements that were specific for my type of cancer. At that time, researching such things was easy to do because censorship had not yet begun. Mindset is also an important aspect of healing because you must work on body, mind, and spirit. I was vigilant in all three areas and eliminated toxic things and people from my life to the best of my ability. Louisiana Medicaid dropped me for refusing chemotherapy, so as of now, 20 years later, I have had two thermography scans to monitor how I am doing, and all is well. Although I miss my grandmother with every fiber of my being, it was witnessing the horrendous effects of her treatment that led me to find other ways. Knowing how I respond to medications due to the MTHFR gene mutation, there is no doubt in my mind that I would not have survived those treatments. I went on to have two more miracle babies in 2006 and 2008 and at age 40 finished up my years of having children. Not only that but because of my decision I was able to breastfeed both of them for the entire first year of their lives with only one breast. It is my opinion that toxins are not and never will be the best choice for a healthy body. I give all credit to the Lord above for guiding me every step of the way through my gift of discernment and the ability to determine what was right for me and the strength to see it through to the end which ultimately was the beginning of a new way of thinking.

Sandra Strickland (Denham Springs, Louisiana)

My cancer journey began in 2007 when I found a lump in my left breast. I went to the doctor, and I was diagnosed with Stage 2 Cancer with 2 tumors in my left breast (2 cm and 1 cm). In 2007, I had a mastectomy of my left breast, and they also removed 11 lymph nodes. I had done chemo, but no radiation at that time. After that, I had breast reconstruction done on my left breast. Fast forward to 2016 and a pea sized lump was found on my right breast. I was diagnosed with Stage 1 cancer, and it was contained. I then had my right breast removed and did six weeks of radiation. A year later, in 2017, I tried to have breast reconstruction done on my right breast using the skin and muscle from my back to reconstruct the breast. The reconstruction surgery didn't take, and I got staph infection and almost died. So, I just opted for the silicone prosthesis.

In the beginning of 2021, I kept having pain in my left breast, but I just shook it off for almost a year. Then I ended up getting a cat during that year and this cat was always sniffing or laying on my left breast or on the left side of my body for some reason. I had heard of cats knowing when someone has cancer, they can smell it. By October of 2021, I finally decided to go to the doctor to find out. The doctor had told me that I had fluid on my left breast, so they drained the fluid and then they found cancer again in my left breast. There was also fluid in the lining of my left lung. So, on October 7, 2021, I was diagnosed with Stage 4 cancer of the left breast, lung and diaphragm. The doctor said that there was nothing they could do at that time. The only thing that the doctor said that I could do was take Ibrance to manage the cancer. I took the Ibrance for two weeks in October of 2021, but it made me so violently ill that I couldn't function, so I stopped taking it.

At around that time, my friend Amber had been researching fenbendazole for healing cancer, so she sent me the information. I couldn't afford the protocol at the time, but she sent me the entire fenbendazole protocol for cancer for the first couple of months. In November of 2021, I began taking fenbendazole, serrapeptase, tudca, and turmeric. I also started on the rick Simpson protocol using full extract cannabis oil (FECO) because I had gotten a medical marijuana card to heal cancer. I also started taking a high dose melatonin. I juiced vegetables and also did Epsom salt baths. I took all of this for 11 months after stopping Ibrance. The first three months there was no cancer growth. At the six-month mark, the cancer started going away. By 11 months in, I was declared no evidence of disease (NED) and that was in September of 2022. I dropped a lot of weight while I was doing this protocol, but it leveled out eventually. I never told my doctor anything about what I was doing, but the doctor knew that I was no longer taking Ibrance but doing something else. The doctor realized that the cancer was going away, he said to just keep doing whatever I was doing. I am now on just a maintenance dose of fenbendazole, tudca, serrapeptase, and D3. I watch what I eat, and I don't eat any sweets.

I don't know why I got cancer as it doesn't run in my family, and I have been tested for the cancerous genes, and it always comes up negative. I had a lot of stress and trauma in my life, being in a few marriages to narcissistic, sociopaths which caused me extreme stress and trauma. I also had a lot of stress from taking care of my dad who was sick and then I lost my house in a flood in Louisiana during a bad storm. I honestly think that it is stress and the food supply which causes so many cancers today. It is strange that even through all I have been through, all of the cancer, the surgeries, the barbaric treatments, I was never sad, but I just kept going and pushing through. I owe my healing to God as he brought Amber to my path to show me the fenbendazole protocol.

My advice for anyone who is going through cancer, or any illness, is for you to listen to your body and pay attention to the pain, don't shrug it off. Also, be your own advocate as doctors fail to listen and do your research on alternatives for healing. Have faith in God, keep a positive mindset, and it is helpful if you have a good support system. I truly believe that if God knows you are strong, and you are a warrior, he will use you for his Glory. If God brings you to it, he'll bring you through it.

James B. Hill (Harrison Township, Michigan)

Jim has stage 4 melanoma. It started as a small spot on his left calf four years ago in 2009. He had this surgically removed along with a sentinel lymph node. The next one showed up on his left thigh a year later in 2010 and once again was surgically removed along with another sentinel lymph node. In 2011 a bump developed on his left groin. Because he had had sentinel lymph nodes removed with the first two surgeries, the doctors thought it was scar tissue. A biopsy revealed the cancer had spread to the lymph and 12 nodes were removed, though only one was found to be cancerous. The oncologist recommended Interferon treatment, even though the chances of it working were only 5-7%. We decided it would do more damage than good to the body and turned it down. That oncologist said there was nothing further he could do until other symptoms were presented, so I changed oncologists.

Going to another cancer treatment hospital, I found a caring and compassionate oncologist. She ordered PET and CAT scans and discovered 3 internal tumors, one on and one inside the intestines, and one on his pelvis. With this next surgery, both of the tumors on and in the intestines were completely removed, but the one on the pelvis could only be partially removed. A chemical treatment called Ipilimumab (also known as Ipi or Yervoy) was offered. It is described as a monoclonal antibody. This is a drug that is supposed to help boost the immune system. Not knowing what else to do, he took one of four treatments prescribed. We discovered it could cause damage to the liver and the liver is very important in healing and detoxing the body, so we stopped the treatment. This drug does not cure; it would only extend his life expectancy by a few months.

This is where Gerson Therapy comes in. We were directed to it by several sources and began researching like crazy. We contacted the Clinic and were lucky enough to be accepted and could get in immediately. Jim is very strong and very determined to beat this. Throughout all of his cancer, he has never had any pain and never felt bad. He has a very positive attitude and wants to live to be 100 (he's 67 now).

The Gerson Clinic in Tijuana, Mexico is a wonderful place for people to learn how to heal in a natural way, through diet and detoxing. While we were there, people arrived from all over the world; Peru, Korea, England, Ireland, Ecuador and from all over the U.S as well. All but one patient was there because of cancer. Some had used conventional medicine already and some chose to just do Gerson.

This is very different from conventional treatment, and that takes some getting used to. The doctors and staff take very good care of the patients with fresh organic meals, juices, supplements, castor oil and clay packs for pain and lots of rest. Blood tests are done weekly, and vitals are taken 3 times a day. You also meet with the head doctor every day. The experience for every patient is different, depending on their level of pain and how advanced their condition is. Since Jim is very strong and looks healthy, the Gerson treatment for him was only about getting used to a different diet, learning how to detox and taking different supplements. Various healing reactions are experienced by some, but Jim did not have any. The motto the patients had while we were there was "I am happy, I am healthy, I am healed, I am whole."

We own a yoga studio in Michigan and are surrounded by supportive and loving people. Our friends and family are willing to help in any way we might need them. We also hope to be an example of how natural healing can take place. We have both changed our eating habits, now looking at food as a way to keep the body strong and healthy and in a constant state of healing. Written by his wife; Pat Hill.

John Tod (Ottawa, Canada)

Back in 1997, my then wife was diagnosed with Hairy Cell Leukemia and was told that she would have to have chemotherapy treatments. She was terrified because she had to watch both her mother and aunt die from Cancer. I researched the web for days until I came across a website that explained everything about Essiac, an herbal tea that boosts the immune system to kill the cancer. Other web pages had many testimonials to its use. I decided to buy some and try it, but I did not hold out much hope because how could an herbal tea cure cancer? We prepared it according to directions and I gave her four ounces, three times a day, for six weeks. After the six weeks she had an appointment at the hospital to see how much further the leukemia had spread. They could find no trace of it! Even after they removed the spleen and did an autopsy on it, it still showed no trace of the cancer, and she lived cancer free until April of 2009 when she passed away from emphysema and COPD caused by a life of heavy smoking.

In December of 2009, our cat was diagnosed with a cancerous bone tumor. I had related the above story to my then wife and she said why not try it on the cat. They wanted to amputate the leg and put the cat on chemo. A very expensive treatment and even if it survived it would only have three legs. I called Essiac Canada and asked for advice. They said because of the weight of the cat (7 pounds) we should give the cat 1/2 a capsule in the morning and evening. The only way to get the Essiac into the cat was to mix it with fruit juice and use a syringe to give it to her at the corner of the mouth. After the first week the cat stopped limping, but we continued the treatment for six weeks. After the six weeks we took our cured cat back to the vet and asked for another x-ray. The new x-ray still showed a bump on the bone but other than that the cat was fine. The vet sent the x-rays away to be interpreted by the same Radiologist who did the first interpretation, and the report came back. It blew all of us away, including the vet. The report said, "less evidence of Lyses" (cancerous activity) and that the bone was "remodeling" and the "continued conservative treatment should be continued." We had already stopped the treatment a couple of weeks before and the vet saw no need for further treatment. My four-legged cat is still alive in November of 2012.

Delynn Potter (Conroe, TX)

My name is Delayne, and my twin brother Delynn (45) was diagnosed with Esophageal Cancer in 2010. He had trouble eating and drinking due to pain. He began chemo treatment in July. He refused to eat or drink and began to lose weight. He seemed to give up. I researched natural therapies and learned of Cell Quest from a survivor. I purchased the product, and my brother agreed to take it. In three days, my brother began to eat and drink normally and did so for the rest of his treatment period. Tests showed his tumor had decreased in size by 70%. By the end of his treatments in December, his tumor was gone and only scar tissue remained. He had surgery as a precaution. He drank 4 ounces twice a day with orange juice. He would follow it with Sodium Bicarbonate in water with Molasses. My brother beat his cancer and has no signs of it coming back. He still has issues from the surgery, but they are not cancer related.

Marcia Schaeffer (Madison, WI)

"We are products of our past. We don't have to be prisoners of it."

On December 6th, 2010, I was sitting in UW Hospital, after having 4 needles stuck in my neck. Keegan wasn't talking yet, or really moving much for that matter. 3 months old – how was my brand-new baby supposed to have ANY clue what was happening?

I still remember Dr. Jaume coming in that room with the fellow. He was so quiet when he told me the diagnosis. He spoke quietly, and pretty quickly. It's funny how I can remember that like it was yesterday. To this day, I STILL shake my head at the fact I texted my family to tell them I had cancer - ha - who does that?! I have to laugh though, to honestly see it as that small of an issue that I could just text the information out is crazy to me. My diagnosis was metastatic thyroid cancer to the lymph nodes and lungs, and malignant melanoma. Stage II Thyroid, Stage I Melanoma. It wasn't all fun and games, and it wasn't all lighthearted.

When Dr. Jaume started telling me about the support groups at the hospital, and how papillary thyroid cancer has great results - I lost it. To be honest, I wasn't scared at all, I was pissed off. It was December, and my prior 12 months had been an absolute whirlwind – In February, I had graduated as a Doctor of Chiropractic, and I was SO fired up to go save the world! The weekend before graduation, I got the privilege of marrying a man I am honored to get to call my husband. Then pregnancy – an incredibly happy, healthy one at that! I loved being pregnant, I loved everything about growing our family – granted, everything was happening incredibly quick, for whatever reason, it was welcomed and enjoyed from the start! The days and nights I had spent with Keegan, both of us learning to breastfeed, were another story – I knew it was a requirement for him, but it sure can test you at times! Going through everything to make it comfortable for both of us, it had JUST got to the point of being ok, I didn't cringe every time I fed him, and now I was supposed to give it up. Not a chance! We are so ingrained with what we learn, and what we want is best, sometimes we don't see the immediate situation. When the nurse said "it's your choice - get your baby a good first year of breastfeeding, or don't watch him graduate high school" I knew the point she was making. I still didn't stop breastfeeding.

Surgery would happen on January 3rd - total thyroidectomy and 30 lymph nodes removed. Later we would find out 26 were positive for cancer. My world would once again be rocked in February. Once again, I remember that morning, I was half awake in bed and my phone started vibrating. My eyes flew open, and my gut churned - I had this sinking feeling it was UW Hospital, once again. Sure enough, I answered the phone, and it was the dermatologist, and she said "You don't even know how hard it is for me to say this to you..." Malignant Melanoma.

My strength at that point was gone. No more happy go lucky Marcia. That was the first time I actually got scared. I remember lying in bed, crying. I was SO frustrated! What was going on in my body that made it so toxic? What was happening to me? Was I bound to have to do the chemo and radiation route? That thought didn't stay long, but it did cross my mind once or twice. Unfortunately, it only crossed my mind when well-meaning people that I love very much were scared for me, and only wanted what they thought was best.

Poor Shawn - who signs up for this?! In one year - a marriage, a baby and cancer. He never showed me his fear. We talked a lot about it, and he knew very well my desires - mainly that I was put on this earth, and I have no idea when my time to go is, so I'll do what I can, and if it is meant to be, it is up to me! He has been such a rock through all of this, I can't imagine my life without him - I know I never would have gotten through all of this without his help and let me tell you - we have been through more in 2 years of marriage than would wish on anyone!!

In March, when the CT came back positive for cancer, I was just irritated all over again. I had done zeolite, cesium protocol, and juicing had started. I knew Gerson Therapy was my choice, but we were getting rid of as much cancer as we could. Victim mentality had left my persona, and I was ready to face whatever I had to in order to live my life to the fullest. I made a deal with God. Let me live, let me serve - and I will do so abundantly. My new favorite phrase came to mind "if it is to be, it is up to me"

An almost overwhelming sense of peace took over after that last CT scan. I knew I was going to Mexico. We didn't have the funds and started looking into bank loans. We got accepted for the bank loan. The stress of how we would pay it back got pretty intense, but unknowingly to us, angels are here on earth. We got an interest free loan, and we were on our way to start healing! I knew then there wasn't a doubt that I would kick this thing out of next year. Not a chance it would stick. Was my sense of peace because I learned a lesson I needed to learn? Was I really THAT hardheaded that I needed cancer to make me change my ways? If so, ok, I mean, I would have appreciated it a bit later, but hey, at least it's over, and I can get on to enjoying the rest of my life with a renewed sense of self and honor.

People think I have lived these 18 months in a bubble. Maybe I have. I have been told I am "too happy to have cancer" NEWS FLASH - it ISN'T about what happens to you; it is COMPLETELY about how you respond to what happens to you!! You can choose to live life in a bubble, and constantly think the world will cave in on you, or you can put yourself out there and make a difference. I chose to write a blog for many reasons, one being to keep family and friends updated, but after this year, I also think it was a part of my therapy. I truly believe one of the reasons this cancer graced my life was because I wasn't honest and open when I was younger. I just wanted approval. Quite obviously, that has changed!!

Clichés are so...cliché. But wow, there is no wonder as to why they were told, and why they stick! I am SO honored I was chosen for this cancer, to learn this way, and to take charge of my health and life, physically, mentally, emotionally. I never would have met the people I have met; I wouldn't have the friendships I have, and I wouldn't have the PROFOUND difference in life experiences that I now have. Now, 18 months after I started Gerson Therapy, I have been "cancer free" according to Western Standards for 9 months now. I will never see my life without the juices I now love, and neither will my son or husband.

On September 6th, 2011, about 9 months after my first diagnosis, I was considered "cancer free" no more tumor markers, no more cancer, via Western Standards. But my knowledge over the past year has far surpassed any notion that cancer is just when a tumor is present or not. Cancer is a lifestyle, a way of being, I have learned a lesson I will never forget and will continue to serve with love as many as I can, to spread the word that cancer is no different than a cold or flu, respect nature, and it respects you.

You don't start living until you find your purpose. Some people live their whole lives searching for purpose. Everything DOES happen for a reason, and I am humbled and honored to learn the true strength and power the human mind and body can comprehend.

www.springcreekfamilychiro.com

Chapter 22
Conclusion

I pray that you have found this book enlightening and beneficial in your path to health and wellness. I had created the "Defeat Cancer Now" plan to save you the confusion, many hours of research, and to make your journey into wellness an easier one. If you take one thing away from this book, my hope for you is to begin to do your own research and expand your knowledge in the area of alternative treatments.

Do not just take my word for it or the word of your doctor, but please do yourself a favor and increase your knowledge base and make your own decision as to what is the best route for you. Ask questions about western medicine and alternative medicine to intensify your knowledge.

Knowledge is power and the more you know about the various ways of healing cancer and disease, the better off you will be to make an intelligent and informed decision for your own health. In the grand scheme of things, listen to your heart and pray for guidance. God will always lead you in the right direction if you just ask him and remain faithful. "You Can Achieve Optimum Health through God's Pharmacy."

References

Required Disclaimer

1. Exodus 23:25. Life Application Study Bible. New Living Translation. (1988). Illinois: Tyndale House Publishers, Inc.

Chapter 2
Why Are We Getting Sick?

1. Basic Information about Fluoride in Drinking Water. (2012. May 21). Retrieved from United States Environmental Protection Agency Website: http://water.epa.gov/drink/contaminants/basicinformation/fluoride.cfm

2. Group, E. The Dangers of Fluoride. (2009. March 26). Retrieved from Global Healing Center Website http://www.globalhealingcenter.com/natural-health/how-safe-is-fluoride

3. Miller, D. Fluoride Follies (n.d.) Retrieved from Tetrahedron Publishing Group Website http://www.tetrahedron.org/articles/health_risks/fluoride_follies.html

4. Smith, J. (n.d.) What is a GMO. Retrieved from The Institute for Responsible Technology Website www.responsibletechnology.org

5. President's Cancer Panel Warns Public of Chemical Dangers. (n.d.)
Retrieved from Environmental Working Group Website http://www.ewg.org/chemindex/term/510

6. National Drinking Water Database. (2009 December).
Retrieved from Environmental Working Group Website http://www.ewg.org/tap-water/executive-summary

7. Persistent Bioaccumulative and Toxic (PBT) Chemical Program. (n.d.).
Retrieved from Environmental Protection Agency Website http://www.epa.gov/pbt/pubs/ddt.htm

8. Smith, J. State of the Science on the Health Risks of GM Foods (2010 February 15).
Retrieved from Institute for Responsible Technology Website http://www.responsibletechnology.org/docs/145.pdf

9. The Disgusting Symptoms of Agent Orange (Dioxin) Poisoning. (2011. May 9).
Retrieved from Vets Helping Vets Website http://www.myveteran.org/2011/05/agent-orange-symptoms.html

10. National Cancer Act of 1971. (n.d.).
Retrieved from The National Cancer Institute Website http://dtp.nci.nih.gov/timeline/noflash/milestones/M4_Nixon.htm

11. Campbell, C. & Campbell T. (2006).
The China Study. Texas: Benbella Books.

Chapter 3
What Is Cancer?

1. Fatigue and Cancer Fatigue. (n.d.).
Retrieved from Cleveland Clinic Website http://my.clevelandclinic.org/disorders/cancer/hic_cancer-related_fatigue.aspx

2. Characteristics of Benign and Malignant Tumors. (2009. December 11). Retrieved from Health Hype Website http://www.healthhype.com/characteristics-of-benign-and-malignant-tumors.html

3. Simoncini, T. Cancer is a Fungus (n.d.). Retrieved from Cancer is a Fungus Website http://www.cancerisafungus.com/cancer-therapy-chapter-4b.php

4. Budwig, J. (1999). Cancer; The Problem and the Solution. Germany: Nexus Books

5. Budwig, J. (1992). Flax Oil as a True Aid against Arthritis, Heart Infarction, Cancer, and Other Diseases. Canada: Apple Publishing Inc.

6. Cantwell Jr., A. (1983) AIDS: THE MYSTERY AND THE SOLUTION. California: Aries Rising Press.

7. Presentation Speech. The Nobel Prize in Physiology or Medicine (1926). Retrieved from Nobel Prize.org Website http://www.nobelprize.org/nobel_prizes/medicine/laureates/1926/press.html

8. Roland, M. Cancer-A Biophysicists Point of View. (2006. September 4). Retrieved from Digital Recordings Website http://www.digital-recordings.com/publ/cancer.html

9. Campbell, C. & Campbell T. (2006). The China Study. Texas: Benbella Books.

10. From Nobel Lectures. Physiology or Medicine 1922-1941. Elsevier Publishing Company. Amsterdam. (1965). Retrieved from Nobel Prize Website http://nobelprize.org/nobel_prizes/medicine/laureates/1931/warburg-bio.html

Chapter 4
Why You Haven't Heard Of Alternative Methods

1. Griffin, G.E. (n.d.) He who pays the piper; the Creation of the Modern Medical (Drug) Establishment.
Retrieved from Foundation in Truth of Reality Website http://www.sntp.net/fda/piper_griffin.htm

2. Griffin, G.E. (1974).World Without Cancer; The Story of Vitamin B17, part 2.
California: American Media.

3. Campbell, C. & Campbell T. (2006).
The China Study. Texas: Benbella Books.

Chapter 5
A Question of Genetics

1. Campbell, C. & Campbell T. (2006). The China Study. Texas: Benbella Books.

Chapter 6
Detoxification

1. Colbert, D. (2000).
Toxic Relief. Florida: Siloam Press.

2. Herbal Parasite Killing Cleanse. (n.d.).
Retrieved from Dr. Clark's Legacy Website http://www.drhuldaclark.org/herbal-parasite-killing-cleanse/

3. Liver Cleanse. (n.d.).
Retrieved from Dr. Clark's Legacy Website http://www.drhuldaclark.org/liver-cleanse/

4. Coffee Enemas Reverses Cancer; By Waste Removal and Detoxifying. (n.d.).

Treating Cancer Alternatively Website, Retrieved from http://www.treating-cancer- alternatively.com/Coffee-enemas.html

5. What is Candida. (n.d.).

Retrieved from The Candida Diet Website. http://www.thecandidadiet.com/

6. Wilson, L. Coffee Enemas: History & Benefits. (2012. April 21).

Retrieved from Healing AIA Holistic Website http://www.healingaia.com/blog-resources/nutritional-balancing/five-elements-of-nutritional-balancing/detox-protocols/coffee-enemas

7. Cairo, M. & Bishop, M. (2004). Tumour lysis syndrome: new therapeutic strategies and classification.

British Journal of Haematology, 127: 3–11. doi: 10.1111/j.1365-2141.2004.05094.x, Retrieved from Wiley Online Library Website http://onlinelibrary.wiley.com/doi/10.1111/j.1365-2141.2004.05094.x/full

8. Harter Pierce, T. (2000).

Outsmart Your Cancer; Alternative Non-Toxic Treatments That Work. Nevada: Thoughtworks Publishing.

Chapter 7
The Power of Enzymes

1. MacKay D. Research on Bromelain; Nutritional Support for Wound Healing. (2003. November 8).

Retrieved from Bromelain Website http://www.bromelain.net/herbal-remedies/bromelain/research-on-bromelain

2. Murray, M. Pancreatic Enzymes; Key to Powerful Anti-Inflammatory & Immune Support. (n.d.).

Retrieved from My Health My Body Natural Products for Healthy Living Website http://www.myhealthmybody.com/trellis/ADM1745_Pancreatic_Enzymes 3. Mosby's Dental Dictionary, 2nd edition. © 2008 Elsevier, Inc. Retrieved from The Free Dictionary Website http://medical-dictionary.thefreedictionary.com/proteolytic

3. University of Utah Health Sciences (2009. August 18). Does Sugar Feed Cancer?

Retrieved from Science Daily Website http://www.sciencedaily.com/releases/2009/08/090817184539.htm

4. Sugar and Cancer. (n.d.).

Retrieved from Healing Cancer Naturally Website. http://www.healingcancernaturally.com/sugar-and-cancer.html

5. Harter Pierce, T. (2000).

Outsmart Your Cancer; Alternative Non-Toxic Treatments That Work. Nevada: Thoughtworks Publishing.

Chapter 8
The Budwig Protocol

1. Budwig, J. (1952).

The Oil Protein Diet Cookbook. Canada: Apple Publishing.

2. Budwig, J. (2011).

The Budwig Cancer and Coronary Heart Disease Prevention Diet. California: Freedom Press Publishing.

3. Budwig, J. (1999).

Cancer The Problem and the Solution. Germany: Nexus Books.

4. Budwig, J. (1992).

Flax Oil as a True Aid against Arthritis, Heart Infarction, Cancer, and Other Diseases. Canada: Apple Publishing.

5. The Budwig Protocol. (n.d.).

Retrieved from Healing Cancer Naturally Website. http://www.healingcancernaturally.com/budwig_protocol.html

6. The Budwig Diet. (n.d.).

Retrieved from The Cancer Cure Foundation Website. http://www.cancure.org/budwig_diet.htm

7. Johanna Budwig Revisited. (n.d.).

Retrieved from International Wellness Directory Website. http://www.mnwelldir.org/docs/cancer1/budwig.htm

8. Adachi, K. Duke University boasts "new" study on flaxseed and cancer; Excuse me, ever heard of Johanna Budwig? (2001. August 15).

Retrieved from Educate Yourself Website http://educate-yourself.org/fc/dukestudyignorsbudwigwork15aug01.shtml

9. Dr. Johanna Budwig. (n.d.).

Retrieved from Health and Well-Being Website. http://www.lightsv.org/bud1.htm 10. Jenkins, L. Johanna Budwig Biography. (n.d.). Retrieved from Budwig Center Website. http://www.budwigcenter.com/johanna-budwig-biography.php

10. Jenkins, L. Cancer Guide (n.d.).

Retrieved from Budwig Center Website. http://www.budwigcenter.com/downloads/budwig-cancer-guide.pdf

11. The Johanna Budwig Cancer Diet. Discover How Stress Causes Cancer and How to Heal Within. (n.d.).

Retrieved from Alternative Cancer Care Website http://www.alternative-cancer-care.com/Johanna_Budwig_Cancer_Diet.html

12. Cancer; Essentially a problem of right and wrong fats & lack of sunlight. (n.d.).

Retrieved from Healing Cancer Naturally Website. http://www.healingcancernaturally.com/budwig_protocol.html#Budwig%20major%20discovery

13. From Nobel Lectures. Physiology or Medicine 1922-1941. Elsevier Publishing Company. Amsterdam. (1965).

Retrieved from Nobel Prize Website http://nobelprize.org/nobel_prizes/medicine/laureates/1931/warburg-bio.html

14. Fischer, W. (2000).

How to Fight Cancer & Win. Maryland: Agora Health Books.

Chapter 9
Drink Your Vegetables

1. Manheim, J. (n.d.). Juicing vs. Blending.

Retrieved from Healthy Green Drink Website. http://healthygreendrink.com/juicing-vs-blending/

2. Eat Goitrogens in Moderation and that includes Soy and Soya. (n.d.).

Retrieved from Stop the Thyroid Madness website from http://www.stopthethyroidmadness.com/goitrogens/

3. What are Goitrogens and what does it mean to the Hypothyroid. (n.d.).

Retrieved from Hypothyroidism and Diet Information Website. http://www.hypothyroidismdietinfo.com/hypothyroidism-diet/hypothyroidism-diet-what-are-goitrogens.php

4. The Gerson Therapy. (2011. September 16).

Retrieved from Gerson Clinic Website http://www.gerson.org/

5. Walker. N.W. (1970).

Fresh Vegetable and Fruit Juices. Arizona: Norwalk Press.

6. Fischer, W. (2000).
How to Fight Cancer & Win. Maryland: Agora Health Books.

7. Harter Pierce, T. (2000).
Outsmart Your Cancer; Alternative Non-Toxic Treatments That Work. Nevada: Thoughtworks Publishing.

Chapter 10
Apricot Kernels

1. Introduction to The Story of Vitamin B17. (n.d.).
Retrieved from World without Cancer Organization, The Story of Vitamin B17 Website. http://www.worldwithoutcancer.org.uk/introduction.html

2. The Hoax of the "Proven" Cancer Cures. (n.d.).
Retrieved from World without Cancer Organization, The Story of Vitamin B17 Website. Retrieved from http://worldwithoutcancer.org.uk/hoax.html

3. The Answer to Cancer is Known. (n.d.).
Retrieved from Apricots from God Website. http://www.apricotsfromgod.info/

4. Genesis 1:29.
Life Application Study Bible. New Living Translation. Illinois: Tyndale House Publishers, Inc.

5. "The Ultimate Guide to Vitamin B-17 Metabolic Therapy." (2000).
Retrieved from World Without Cancer Website http://worldwithoutcancer.org.uk/FINALGUIDEUKpdfEbook.pdf

6. "The Ultimate Cancer Conspiracy." (n.d.).
Retrieved from Cancer and Biopsy Website http://www.karlloren.com/biopsy/p76.htm

7. Krebs, E. (n.d.). "The Nature of Cancer."
Retrieved from http://www.whale.to/cancer/krebs.html

8. Krebs, E. (1964). "The Nitrilosides in Plants and Animals; Nutritional and Therapeutic Implications." John Beard Memorial Foundation.
Retrieved from The Robert Cathey Research Source http://users.navi.net/~rsc/nitrilo1.htm

9. Griffin, E. (1974).
World Without Cancer; The Story Of Vitamin B17. California: American Media.

10. Harter Pierce, Tanya (2000).
Outsmart Your Cancer; Alternative Non-Toxic Treatments That Work. Nevada: Thoughtworks Publishing.

11. Fischer, W. (2000).
How to Fight Cancer & Win. Maryland: Agora Health Books.

Chapter 11
pH Balance & Nutrition

1. "The Cause of Disease; PH Imbalance." Lesson 18. (n.d.).
Retrieved from Natural Health School Website http://www.naturalhealthschool.com/acid-alkaline.html_

2. Young, R. & Young, S. (2002).
The pH Miracle; Balance Your Diet, Reclaim Your Health. New York: Warner Books.

3. "Alkalize Your Body pH to Restore Good Health." (n.d.).
Retrieved from Balance pH Diet Website http://www.balance-ph-diet.com

4. McEvoy, M. "Acid & Alkaline Nutrition: Shattering the Myths." (n.d.).
Retrieved from Metabolic Healing Website http://metabolichealing.com/education/articles/acid-and-alkaline-nutrition-shattering-the-myths/

5. Timberlake, K. (2006).
Chemistry; An Introduction to General, Organic, and Biological Chemistry. Ninth Edition. Pearson Education.

6. Widmaier, E., Hershel, R., & Strang, K. (2006).
Human Physiology; The Mechanisms of Body Function. Tenth Edition. McGraw Hill Higher Education.

7. Mercola, J. "If You Fall For This Water Fad, You Could Do Some Major Damage." (2010. September 11).
Retrieved from Mercola Website http://articles.mercola.com/sites/articles/archive/2010/09/11/alkaline-water-interview.aspx

8. Howell, E. (2003). "Is Your Body Demanding Food Enzymes?"
Retrieved from LifeSources Inc. Website http://www.life-sources.com/pages/Is-Your-Body-Demanding-Food-Enzymes%3F.html

9. Baum, J. "Symptoms That the Body Is Too Alkaline." (2011. March 28).
Retrieved from Livestrong Website http://www.livestrong.com/article/154113-symptoms-that- the-body-is-too-alkaline/

10. Sellers, K. "Can Your Body's pH be Too Alkaline?" (2008. April 24).
Retrieved from Natural News Website http://www.naturalnews.com/023097_alkaline_water_body.html

11. Cohen, M. "Emmanuel Revici M.D.; Innovator in Nontoxic Cancer Chemotherapy. (n.d.).
Retrieved from Revici Medical Website http://www.revicimedical.com/About_Dr_Revici.htm

Chapter 13
Epidermal Growth Factor Receptor

1. Reck, Martin & Gutzmer, R. (2010). Management of the Cutaneous side effects of therapeutic epidermal growth factor receptor inhibition. Onkologie, 33.

Retrieved from Bio Med Search Website http://www.biomedsearch.com/nih/Management-cutaneous-side-effects-therapeutic/20838065.html

2. Cutaneous Side Effects Associated With Targeted Therapy. (2009. November 5).

Retrieved from OncUview TV, Oncology News, Education, and Information Website.http://www.oncuview.tv/SymptomManagement/tabid/67/articleType/ArticleView/articleId/7/Cutaneous-Side-Effects-Associated-With-Targeted-Therapy.aspx

3. Cancer Growth Blockers. (n.d.).

Retrieved from Cancer Research UK Website http://www.cancerhelp.org.uk/about-cancer/treatment/biological/types/cancer-growth-blockers

4. EGFR. (n.d.).

Retrieved from National Cancer Institute at the National Institutes of Health Dictionary of Cancer terms http://www.cancer.gov/dictionary/?CdrID=44397

5. Kuriyan, J. Researchers Learn How Epidermal Growth Factor Receptor is Activated. (2006. June 15).

Retrieved from Howard Hughes Medical Institute Website. http://www.hhmi.org/news/kuriyan20060615.html

6. Kuriyan, J. Structural Biology of Cell Signaling and DNA Replication. (2012. May 30).

Retrieved from Howard Hughes Medical Institute Website. http://www.hhmi.org/research/investigators/kuriyan.html

7. Murray, M. Pancreatic Enzymes; Key to Powerful Anti-Inflammatory & Immune Support. (n.d.).

Retrieved from My Health My Body Natural Products for Healthy Living Website. http://www.myhealthmybody.com/trellis/ADM1745_Pancreatic_Enzymes

8. Benefits of Bromelain. (n.d.).

Retrieved from Bromelain Website. http://www.bromelain.net/herbal-remedies/bromelain/benefits-of-bromelain

9. Pancreatic Cancer, Proteolytic Enzyme Therapy and Detoxification. (1999. November).

Retrieved from Dr. Gonzalez Website Clinical Pearls Newsletter http://www.dr- gonzalez.com/clinical_pearls.htm

10. "Stages and Types of Cancer" (n.d.).

Retrieved from Family Doctor Website. http://familydoctor.co.uk/info/stages-types-of-breast-cancer

Chapter 16
The Navarro Urine Test

1. Information & HCG Urine Test. (n.d.).

Retrieved from Navarro Medical Clinic Website. www.navarromedicalclinic.com

2. Cantwell, A. (1983).

AIDS; The Mystery & The Solution. California: Aries Rising Press.

3. Harter Pierce, T. (2000).
Outsmart Your Cancer; Alternative Non-Toxic Treatments That Work. Nevada: Thoughtworks Publishing.

4. Fischer, W. (2000).
How to Fight Cancer and Win. Maryland: Agora Health Books.

Chapter 17
Preventing Cancer & Other Diseases

1. Fife, B. (2005).
Coconut Cures. Colorado: Piccadilly Books, Ltd.

Chapter 18
Faith in God & Healing Scriptures

1. Scripture taken from the New King James Version.

Calling for Your Input

I would love to read your comments on what you thought of the book. Was it easy to understand, have you started the "Defeat Cancer Now" plan and how has it helped you? All comments may end up on the webpage, Facebook page, or future publications of Lake Front Publishing and Tamara St. John.

After reading this book, are you left with any questions? If so, please send an email through my website contact form so I can make the proper revisions for a future edition.

I would also like to include your testimonial, if you used alternative treatments to heal your cancer naturally, even if you started with western medicine, I would love to hear from you. Your testimonial may end up in a future edition of the book or on my website. Please send your testimonial through my contact form on my webpage.

Thank you so much and Blessings to all.

Tamara St. John
www.Tamarastjohn.com

www.ingramcontent.com/pod-product-compliance
Lightning Source LLC
Chambersburg PA
CBHW060947050426
42337CB00052B/1633

* 9 7 9 8 9 9 2 4 6 7 3 0 7 *